Smart Exercise

BOOKS BY COVERT BAILEY

Fit or Fat?
The Fit-or-Fat Target Diet
The New Fit or Fat
Smart Exercise

BOOKS BY COVERT BAILEY
AND LEA BISHOP

Fit-or-Fat Target Recipes
The Fit-or-Fat Woman

BOOKS BY COVERT BAILEY
AND RONDA GATES

Smart Eating

Smart Exercise

Burning Fat, Getting Fit

COVERT BAILEY

HOUGHTON MIFFLIN COMPANY

Boston • New York

For information about permission to reproduce selections from
this book, write to Permissions, Houghton Mifflin Company,
215 Park Avenue South, New York, New York 10003.

For information about this and other Houghton Mifflin
trade and reference books and multimedia products, visit
The Bookstore at http://www.hmco.com/trade.

Library of Congress Cataloging-in-Publication Data

Bailey, Covert
Smart exercise : burning fat, getting fit / Covert Bailey
p.   cm.
Includes index.
ISBN 0-395-66114-5 (pbk.)
1. Exercise. 2. Physical fitness. I. Title
GV481.B2356 1994   94-1667
613.7'1 — dc20   CIP

Printed in the United States of America

Book design by Robert Overholtzer

QUM 10 9 8 7 6 5 4 3 2 1

———————

The cartoons in this book were created by Lynn Garnica,
whose ability to make fun when I get too serious is most
refreshing. Concepts that required paragraphs of explanation were captured in her drawings, using no words at all.

*This book is dedicated
to the best man I know,*

GRANT COVERT BAILEY

Lea Bishop

The Greeks had their gods and goddesses who lived with them on earth but were so special that even kings and queens felt like ordinary mortals. I know that these beings were not simply in the Greeks' imaginations because Zeus sent one down to me, a golden-haired goddess who put her magic on every page you are about to read. She won't put her name on our books, and she turns away from recognition. If this book helps you live a better life, perhaps dramatically, you can thank my goddess. She's just an unassuming blond with a steel-trap mind who hides on a farm somewhere in Oregon. Respected but never understood, cherished but never captured.

Contents

2. How Muscle Works

*Even the cheapest car comes with an owner's manual.
What a shame that our magnificent Porsche-quality bodies
don't! I hope the following "owner's manual" hasn't
been delivered too late.*

3. Metabolism

People often say, "My metabolism is slowing down."
What in the world are they talking about!!!

4. Exercise Basics

This section is a "how to" that will rescue you from all
the "how to" books.

5. Training

This is the section that fat people might skip, thinking
that it's not for them. Don't skip it! Most of the best stuff
we know about getting rid of fat comes from research
on athletes and their training.

6. Swimming and Walking

People ask more questions about walking and swim-
ming than about any other exercise. Maybe it's
because everybody knows how to do them, or maybe
it's because they are the refuge activities of people
so out of shape that every other activity looms
as unpleasant.

7. Before Exercise — and After

8. Measuring Your Own Fat and Fitness

You can spend lots of dollars at fancy clinics getting fancy tests, but nothing beats self-measurement. Home tests let you set your own goals — the best motivation for high achievement.

9. Diet Tricks for Performance

Of all the dietary manipulations that have been foisted on athletes, only the ones listed below are worthy of discussion. Let the energy bars, vitamin supplements, amino acids, and pep pills remain with the hucksters who started promoting them.

10. Sweating and Dehydration

11. How to Make More Muscle

You don't have to be a bodybuilder to want more muscle. Muscle does so much for you, it pays to have a lot of it.

12. The Payoff

You could replace all the good information in this book with vigorous sport. Just get involved, and the benefits will roll in automatically!

1

Fitness Equals Health

Covert's Prejudice

Before you read my book you have a right to know my prejudice. Ever since I was a little kid I've noticed that fit people can
do things that unfit people can't. My prejudice is that exercise,
especially sports exercise, can cure almost anything. We're born
with a fabulous machine that is able to repair itself almost like
magic. All you have to do is exercise, and your machine gets
healthier. Imagine owning a car that tuned itself up every time
you drove it! Your wonderful body machine will run better and
better the more you exercise it. I think exercise can cure almost
everything.

Of course "everything" is an exaggeration, but let me give
you an example. I've been asked, "Can you prove that a fit
person's broken bones will heal quicker than those of someone
who isn't fit?" If you read the research, you won't be able to
find enough information to prove it one way or the other. But
think about this. If a really fit guy gets a broken leg, how does
he handle it? He hops around on the other leg, doesn't he? A fat
person with a broken leg hobbles. He moves very slowly and
carefully because he's afraid he's going to fall down and break
the other leg. Fit people deal with a broken leg as a challenge
— a new sport.

I had a bad accident about seven years ago when I fell off a
three-wheeled motorcycle. I broke seven ribs and my hipbone.
Sure I hurt. I was on all kinds of drugs for about three days, and
I was pretty useless for another three. But by the seventh day,
I was outdoors on my crutches, playing. Instead of making me

bitter and angry, my injury became an interesting challenge. How could I get through doors, drive a car, maneuver through a turnstile on crutches? Before long my kids and I were seeing if we could walk around the kitchen on my crutches without letting our feet touch the floor. In two weeks I was out playing Frisbee on one foot. I couldn't run, I had to hop around, but I was playing Frisbee just weeks after a serious accident. Am I super special? No. I'm just like most fit people.

Think of the benefits I gained from my active approach. First, I was having fun, so I was happy. Second, by hopping around on one leg, I got a cross-training effect. Later I'll discuss cross training in more detail, but for now just remember that if you work the muscles of one leg, there is a tendency for your other leg to maintain fitness. Third, I maintained my balance and agility despite having a cast on my leg and hip.

Here's another thing to think about. When you're fit, you're able to rest while being active; that is, what looks like exercise to a fat person may be rest for a fit person. A fit person who is injured or sick spends less time recuperating in bed than someone who isn't fit; and as any doctor can tell you, patients who are on their feet recover more quickly than patients who are flat on their backs in bed.

Can I absolutely prove that a fit person's broken bone heals faster than a fat person's broken bone? No! The actual healing time may be the same, but the fit person, because of the way she lives, will be way ahead once the bone has healed. The fat, unfit person, struggling along with a broken leg, won't be ready for normal activities when the bone has healed because his muscles will have wasted — even if the healing time is the same.

> ### "Can you prove that fit people live longer?"

Similarly, the question "Can you prove that fit people live longer?" is extremely difficult to answer. The research is subject to all kinds of interpretations, but to argue about it misses the point. Fit people, because of all the things they do in life, probably do live longer. Fit people, when they are seventy years old, hike and ski in the mountains. Their blood flows easily because it is thin, their red blood cell count is high, their lungs are healthy, they have strong hearts. They are stronger than unfit people in every way. They withstand trauma and disease far better. So can I prove that fitness itself makes them live longer? No. It's easier to show that *lack* of fitness makes you live *shorter*.

Fit people who play sports are much less likely to spend money on illegal drugs; they don't need them. If all Americans got into sports, and exercise, the government wouldn't have to spend so much money policing drugs. Fit people don't smoke cigarettes, so they're less likely to get cancer. They aren't fat, so they have fewer heart attacks. On the job they have less "down" time from colds and flus, which reduces their own medical expenses and the costs to their employers. Suppose I had been someone's employee when I broke my ribs and hip. My boss would have had to pay me for only about six days of sick time. He wouldn't have had to pay for physical therapy — I did my own! A fat, out-of-shape person would have said, "I can't get from my car to the office," or, "I can't negotiate the stairs." The point is, fit people need less medical care, less time in the hospital, and less time away from work. Fit people are cheap to have around.

Wow — at the rate I'm going, I believe I can come up with a good argument for curing the national debt with exercise!

Even metabolism, that technical-sounding word that nobody understands, is altered by exercise. If you believe your excess fat is caused by faulty metabolism, let me enlighten you — even that problem can be "cured" by exercise. Metabolism isn't as mysterious as it seems. Later on I'll show you a new way to look at metabolism, what you have to do to change it, and how *huge* the effect of exercise is upon it.

This book is not about claims I can't prove. Every statement has been proven by good research. My focus is mainly on measurable physical changes that take place as a result of exercise. I don't go into the psychological advantages of exercise very much, not because they're unimportant, but because they're so subjective. We all somehow sense that exercise is "good for the soul," but how can we prove it? For instance, I talk a lot about walking because it's such a common activity. After I discuss the good and the bad points about walking as exercise, you may conclude that walking isn't that great, but you'd be missing the point. Think about how high you feel after a walk in the moonlight with a good friend. The emotional impact of a good walk on a beautiful evening goes far beyond the physiological impact of walking.

The psychological benefits of any exercise go way beyond the measurable physiological effects. People who are involved in sports are harder to ruffle. Everyday trials and tribulations seem petty after you've been knocked down on the basketball court a few times. And after you've missed some easy layup shots, you aren't irate when the paper boy misses your front step. Little things just don't get to you. In competitive sports, players love to trade insults. Then, when they're off the court, they can laugh about the other little insults in life. These are the psychological benefits of exercise — hard to prove, hard even to discuss, and yet so important. As I say — exercise can cure almost anything.

At a recent party, a medical doctor with a good sense of humor gave us all some sample pills. They tasted very sweet and looked suspiciously like M&M's. He insisted that each one of us would feel better if we took his pills *if* we followed the directions carefully:

> Take two pills with a glass of water immediately after a half hour of aerobic exercise.

We have named these magic pills "King Muscle Pills." I'd like to send you some, but they haven't been released by the FDA, approved by the surgeon general, or sanctioned by the American Medical Association.

But read on — I'll show you how you can get them.

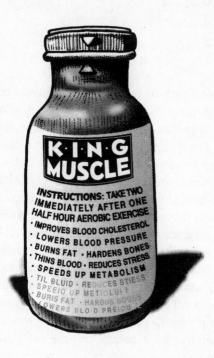

King Muscle!

Exercise makes demands on every organ in the body. The liver responds to exercise by producing glycogen more efficiently. The pancreas responds by fine-tuning its regulation of insulin and glucose. The lungs and heart deliver more oxygen. The circulatory system builds more capillaries. The level of LDL cholesterol in the blood drops, and the level of HDL cholesterol goes up. Even bones respond to exercise by becoming denser.

And, of course, muscle itself responds to exercise. The mitochondria that produce adenosine triphosphate (ATP) enlarge and increase. Its specialized oxidative enzymes increase twofold. With more mitochondria and oxidative enzymes, the muscles learn to burn more and more fat. They become fat-burning machines, and you become a better butter burner.

Muscle comprises 40 percent of a man's weight and 30 percent of a woman's. That means muscle can demand a lot of attention from the other tissues in the body. Muscles at rest are like a car idling at a stoplight. While the light is red, they burn only a few calories, but once it turns green, they burn a tremendous amount of fuel. Most of the time, our muscles are just idling. But they have to maintain an energy system that is *capable* of taking off at any moment.

Muscle is the only tissue that can go from zero to sixty in thirty seconds. The difference between its metabolism at rest and its metabolism at work is extreme. Our other systems aren't like that. Whether you're sleeping or working on a complex physics problem, your brain metabolism doesn't change very much. And the liver, though it is a highly metabolic tissue involved in hundreds of chemical processes, can't increase its metabolism a hundredfold in thirty seconds.

> **Muscle demands that every tissue in the body race to obey its commands.**

Faced with responsibility, muscles become highly demanding. "Hey, fuel pump [heart]! Get some gas down here! You, carburetor lungs! Open up your alveoli and bronchial tubes and get me some air! Can't you see I'm doing sixty-five on the freeway?" Muscle demands that every tissue in the body race to obey its commands.

Now, combine the fact that we are made largely of muscles and the fact that muscles have unique energy needs, and you can begin to see why muscle is at the "heart" of metabolism, your need for calories, and health itself. This is obviously an "exercise is good for you" book. I want people to stop thinking that diet is so important or that one particular organ is at the root of their problems. It's time to tune up the engine! King Muscle rules!

How Is Fitness Measured?

Running is not only a natural human activity and an integral part of many sports, it gives us the most accurate way to measure fitness — the oxygen uptake test. This test involves running to your maximum on a treadmill. The speed and incline of the treadmill are gradually increased until you're running at breakneck speed, gasping for breath, wishing you had never heard of Covert Bailey and the oxygen uptake test. Off to the side, a medic waits with resuscitating paddles in case you pass out. (Naturally the test is voluntary.) Sounds like fun, doesn't it? Actually, it's expensive, time-consuming, and, as you can guess, potentially dangerous.

For one minute during this maximum effort, we measure the amount of oxygen that disappears inside your body. If oxygen, a gas, goes in and doesn't come out, why don't you blow up? Obviously, it's because the oxygen is metabolized into other products. To get a high score on the oxygen uptake test, you have to have a healthy heart, lungs, and blood to absorb and transport oxygen, coupled with fit muscles that can combine the oxygen with sugar and fat to produce energy.

Since the test measures the amount of oxygen your body uses, you might ask, "Is this a lung test?" Or you might think it's a running test. Actually, it is neither; it is a "whole-body" test that measures the efficiency of heart, lungs, blood, and most of the other physiological functions.

Your ability to use oxygen when your body is working at its maximum is directly related to the number of calories you

burn. If you use lots of oxygen when you run you are, by definition, using lots of calories. An out-of-shape person who gasps
and puffs during exercise is not using lots of oxygen. Her body
wants it, she breathes it in, but because her absorption and
transportation systems are poor, most of the oxygen is puffed
right back out. The oxygen uptake test tells us how much of
that oxygen you're breathing in is actually being used.

> **Your ability to use oxygen when
> your body is working at maximum
> is directly related to the number
> of calories you burn.**

We realize now that this test measures not just fitness but
total body health as well. In other words, as the body's ability
to use oxygen improves, physical fitness increases — and you
become healthier.

Having a high rate of oxygen uptake means:

- lower blood pressure
- better heat regulation
- stronger tendons and ligaments
- thicker cartilage
- larger muscles
- greater blood volume
- more hemoglobin
- less body fat
- denser bones
- more efficient lungs
- heart pumps more blood with each stroke
- more oxygen extracted from the blood
- more capillaries
- lower heart rate

Oxygen Uptake and Performance

In the early days of testing, the results of oxygen uptake tests were reported in liters of oxygen per minute. The fitter the person, the more liters he used, and the higher his performance on the test. But describing oxygen uptake in that manner did not take into account differences in body size. I use many more liters of oxygen than my twelve-year-old son simply because I'm bigger than he is — but he is much fitter than I am. Reporting our oxygen uptake in liters leads to the false conclusion that I am fitter than my son. To remedy this error, the test is now based on how much oxygen a person uses *per pound* (or, more commonly, per kilogram) *of body weight*. Thus, the term that describes oxygen uptake is "milliliters per kilogram per minute," and the symbol used is $\dot{V}O_2$ max. The V stands for volume, the O_2 for oxygen, and the little dot over the V represents a unit of time. A person who has a $\dot{V}O_2$ max of 40 uses 40 milliliters of oxygen per kilogram of weight per minute.

$\dot{V}O_2$ max readings range from a low of 15 to a high of 70. People who get $\dot{V}O_2$ max readings of 15 are more than incredibly out of shape — they are probably sick. At the other end of the range, a reading of 70 means you're an Olympic athlete. At $\dot{V}O_2$ max 70, athletes run four-minute miles. Race horses, tested in the same way but on bigger treadmills, get double the $\dot{V}O_2$ max — 140 — and can run a mile in two minutes — twice as fast.

Changes in oxygen uptake follow a curve of diminishing returns. If you're unfit, a small improvement in your $\dot{V}O_2$ max will mean a big improvement in performance. The sedentary person should find this encouraging because with very little effort, he can improve dramatically.

The fat guy can improve his fitness quicker than the fit guy.

If you look at the graph on the next page, you'll see that there's only a small increase in $\dot{V}O_2$ max when a person reduces his one-mile running time from thirty minutes to twenty. A tremendous improvement in performance shows up as only a small increase in oxygen uptake. At the other end of the graph, we see that when you reduce running time from six minutes to four minutes, the change in $\dot{V}O_2$ max is very large. When you're very fit, small improvements in performance require incredible changes in the body's ability to use oxygen.

It's important to note that there is a breaking point to the curve on the graph. When the one-mile running time is somewhere between ten and fifteen minutes, the curve makes a sharp upward turn. This bend in the curve represents the $\dot{V}O_2$ max set point and a distinct change in the physiological effects of exercise. Going beyond this point improves fitness and health, but the return on your effort becomes smaller and smaller as you work harder and harder.

The curve shown here applies to most men. The curve for women is similar but a little farther to the left; because of their smaller size and smaller muscle mass, women get the same health and fitness benefits from running a mile slightly slower than men.

Do higher readings for men mean that men are fitter than women? Men do have more muscle, and it's the amount of active, working muscle that determines how much oxygen is used. If men have more muscle, they're going to use more oxygen. However, if we could measure oxygen uptake per pound of *active* muscle, we'd find no difference between men and women.

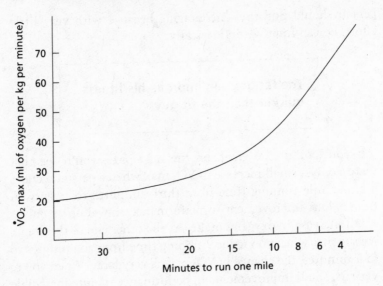

Female muscle uses oxygen just as efficiently as male muscle. Measuring oxygen uptake per pound of active muscle isn't practical because that muscle still has to lug around the rest of the body. Women simply have less muscle and, usually, more fat. Thus, when $\dot{V}O_2$ max per pound of *total* body weight is compared, women tend to have lower $\dot{V}O_2$ max measurements.

Before my male readers get too smug about this, they need to remember that the difference is due in large part to differences in body size and composition. If a woman and a man are equal in performance, they are also equal in $\dot{V}O_2$ max, body composition, maximum heart rate, respiratory exchange ratio, and other indices of fitness. In other words, a woman can be just as fit as a man if their size and muscle-to-fat ratios are the same.

2

How Muscle Works

Even the cheapest car comes with an owner's manual. What a shame that our magnificent Porsche-quality bodies don't! I hope the following "owner's manual" hasn't been delivered too late.

Our Obsession with Fat

Fat: The Primary Fuel

How Fats Move Around

How Muscles Use Fat

What Is an Enzyme?

Fat and Sugar Storage — the Gas Tanks

The Krebs Cycle

Lactic Acid

Ketosis

Emaciated Runners

Fat People Are Sugar Burners

The Exercise Flush

Our Obsession with Fat

Americans are so obsessed with their desire to get rid of body fat that they blame the fat itself. "Fat is terrible!" they say. "I hate fat! Why do I have all this fat?" The truth is that fat is the most efficient gas tank ever designed.

We can make fat out of almost anything we eat. All the carbohydrate in bread, pasta, and potatoes, if it's in excess of what the body needs, can be turned into fat. If we eat more protein than we need, the liver converts it into fat. And we all know that eating too much fat just makes us fatter.

The liver can convert bread, carrots, avocados, potatoes — you name it — into fat. It's actually miraculous! Let's invent a car engine that can turn everything we put into the gas tank to gasoline. Put in avocados and the engine simply converts the avocados into gas. Put in hamburger and our beautiful car converts it into gasoline. Wouldn't that be fabulous? People would respect such a wonderful invention.

> **"Why did God make us have fat?"**

The human machine is just as wonderful. It can convert almost anything you put in your mouth into fat. If your gas tanks are bulging, don't blame the gas tank and don't fault the fabulous fuel-making system. Instead, ask, "Why did God make us this way?" It's as if God said, "Today I am going to design an upright running machine. I've designed foxes, coyotes, deer, and

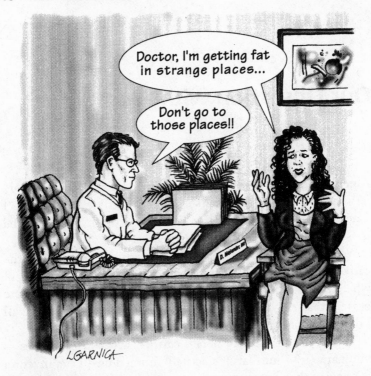

antelope, all of which run fantastically well. But now I want to design a creature that can run on two feet so that the other two feet can be used to hold things. I need to design a special fuel system for this creature since it's only going to have two legs to run on. Its fuel tank must be so perfectly distributed over its body that it won't tip over frontward or backward. I'm going to design this creature so that anything it eats can be converted into its primary fuel."

By now you should be saying, "Holy smokes! I didn't realize that fat is our primary fuel!" I want you to stop blaming your fat! That's where most of the energy comes from when you run, play tennis, or dance. Show some respect for your unbelievably efficient primary-fuel-producing, storing, and burning machine. Instead of going on bizarre diets whose entire intent is to pervert the system God gave you, learn how to use this fuel.

Fat: The Primary Fuel

I have a friend who likes to barbecue on his back deck. He puts charcoal in the grill, squirts some lighter fluid on the charcoal, and throws a match on it. The lighter fluid goes "BOOM," but somehow his charcoal never starts burning. So he squirts more lighter fluid, lights another match, and watches it blow up again while his wife and I make fun of him. He makes frequent trips to the store for more lighter fluid. One day his wife commented, "Charlie's charcoal grill runs on lighter fluid."

In a way, muscle is like that grill. Muscle burns both fat and sugar: the sugar burns instantly like lighter fluid, yielding only a small amount of energy, but the fat continues to burn for a long, long time, like charcoal once it gets started. You get lots more calories, or energy, from a fat molecule than you do from a sugar molecule. When you're playing active sports you may run out of sugar; you never run out of fat.

We now know that even people who are starving never, never, never use up all of their body fat. This may surprise you, since starving or anorexic people look so emaciated, but there is fat even on the bodies of people who weigh only seventy-five pounds. They look like skeletons when they die because they lose so much muscle, but autopsies show that they still have ten or fifteen pounds of fat hidden inside. These people do not, in fact, *starve* to death.

Nobody in the history of the earth has ever actually starved to death. At some point during starvation, as the body runs out of glucose it starts using protein for fuel (see the chapter "Emaciated Runners"). In the process of burning protein, it taps the immune system antibodies, which are proteins. Starving people become highly susceptible to bacteria and viruses; they die of infectious diseases precipitated by lack of protein in their bodies.

> **People worry too much about vitamins, proteins, and carbohydrates — it's FAT that runs the body.**

Like starving people, those who are very fit occasionally have lighter-fluid problems. During long, rigorous sports events their muscles run out of sugar. When that happens, their energy drops abruptly because the burning of fat, triggered by sugar's spark, has ceased. Athletes think they run out of energy because their sugar has run out, but in reality, they have plenty of "fat energy" left but no way to draw from it. They constantly look for ways to store more sugar in their muscles, mistakenly thinking that sugar is their primary fuel. But it is only the starter fluid; fat is the primary fuel.

How Fats Move Around

I wish it were as easy to explain how fat travels in blood as it is to talk about protein and carbohydrates. We eat an incredible variety of proteins, which all end up in the blood as simple amino acids. And the carbohydrates in potatoes, bread, or chocolate pudding all turn into blood glucose. But the fats we eat, which go through the same digestive processes — saliva, stomach acid, and pancreatic enzymes — don't reduce to a simple one-word end product. Instead we get fatty acids, monoglycerides, triglycerides, high-density cholesterol, low-density cholesterol, and a few other tongue twisters. Is it any wonder no one can understand the research reports?

In any case, it's the fatty acids that I want to talk about. Fatty acid molecules are extremely small compared to triglycerides and cholesterol — and they are highly mobile. It's easy for fatty acids to pass through semipermeable membranes, the porous walls of capillaries and cells. They can move out of the bloodstream into a muscle cell to be burned for energy. If the muscle cell says, "I'm not exercising right now," they move back out into the blood again and travel to a fat cell for storage. Because they are so mobile, they are sometimes called *free* fatty acids.

Triglycerides and cholesterol make up the bulk of the fats in the bloodstream. They tend to build up on the inside of coronary arteries and are associated with heart attack, stroke, and diabetes. These are the fats that physicians measure to give us an indication of our risk of having a heart attack.

Free fatty acids, on the other hand, don't deposit on anything. They're moving too quickly, zooming around looking for an exercising muscle. These highly mobile fat molecules make up less than 1 percent of the fats in blood. They are not associated with heart attacks or other cardiovascular disease, but they are important for two reasons:

1. They are the basic fuel for energy.
2. They make us fat.

If we don't use fatty acids for fuel, we store them you-know-where.

> **Fat seems to sit on your hips, immobile, forever, but believe me, it's released immediately if you know the right tricks!**

Even after they're stored, fatty acids don't stay still for long. They readily leave their fat depots, travel through the bloodstream looking for a muscle that needs energy, and, if no muscle needs them, go on to another fat depot. Free fatty acids are in constant flux, sometimes being deposited, sometimes being released from a fat depot, sometimes going to a muscle cell to be burned. All that moving around has only one purpose — to be available for energy.

When they hang out in a fat cell, fatty acids like to bond together in triplets. In this form they are called *tri*-glycerides. All the fat stored in your body is fatty acids in the triglyceride form. Your "beer belly" is nothing more than a big chunk of triglycerides. As the fat depots get bigger, some triglycerides spill out into the bloodstream. When your doctor says your triglycerides are too high, it's his medical way of telling you you're getting too fat.

Triglycerides do two things; they sit around in fat depots, and they're disassembled back into fatty acids when the muscles need fuel. If you can teach your body to metabolize fatty acids, your triglyceride stores will diminish.

How Muscles Use Fat

Whether you're sitting or running, your muscles burn two kinds of fuel at the same time — sugar and fat. Seventy percent of the energy — or calories — that muscles need comes from fat, while only thirty percent comes from sugar. These percentages are reversed when you are exercising very intensely, but that kind of high level doesn't last very long so, overall, fat remains the predominant fuel.

The diagram here shows sugar in the bloodstream on its way to a muscle cell. Blood sugar, more properly called glucose, trickles into the muscle cells along with fatty acids. Inside the cell the two fuels are taken apart by little proteins called enzymes, which release the energy. Since fatty acid molecules are considerably larger than glucose molecules, they release more energy. After the enzymes have done their work, all that's left is carbon dioxide and water. It's similar to burning logs in a fireplace. You can put a tiny log (glucose) and a big log (fat) in your fireplace, and if you can get the darn things going, they will both burn to ashes. In this analogy, the ashes would be carbon dioxide and water.

But unlike the fire in the fireplace, which will go out abruptly if the oxygen supply is cut off, some burning can take place in muscle cells even when the air supply is shut off. Glucose in a muscle can be half burned with no oxygen present; this is called anaerobic burning. When we run so fast that we're out of breath, the muscle also gets "out of breath" and extinguishes its fires — except for the anaerobic burning of glucose.

How the Muscle Makes Energy

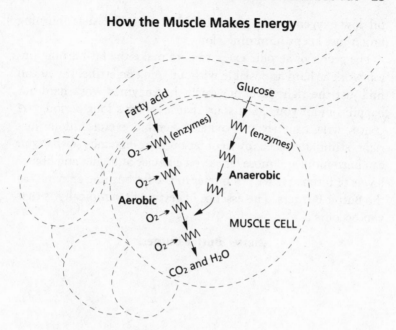

More typically, muscle burns fatty acids and glucose at the same time. The key here is that the burning of fat, and part of the burning of glucose, *requires oxygen,* which is what the word "aerobic" means. A muscle functions aerobically when it has enough oxygen so that the fat-burning enzymes are working as well as the sugar-burning enzymes.

> **The fat-burning enzymes go on strike when you exercise too hard.**

Now comes the fun part. Think of the enzymes that burn fat molecules as a labor union of highly specialized workers. This union tends to go on strike a lot, especially when there is not enough oxygen. Your muscles may be begging for more energy during a fast run, but the fat-burning union, hating such stressful low-oxygen work, goes out on strike. The sugar-burning union just keeps humming along.

The secret of aerobic exercise is to make the fat-burning union work as hard as possible without going on strike. If you can find just the right level at which the enzymes work hard but happily, and if you can sustain that level for a long period, THE UNION WILL HIRE MORE WORKERS. Aerobic exercise, done just right, stimulates the growth of fat-burning enzymes so that you can burn more and more fat as you exercise at higher and higher levels of intensity. We often refer to the fat-burning enzymes as the Butter Burners. The essence of getting fit aerobically is that you become a

Better Butter Burner.

What Is an Enzyme?

One of Bill Cosby's first routines was a conversation between Noah and God concerning the construction of the ark. God tells Noah exactly how long and how wide the ark should be and how many animals it should hold, and after each instruction, Noah says, "Right!" Finally, when God is finished, Noah asks, "What's an ark?"

It occurred to me that my readers might be in the same boat (yes, pun intended). I've talked about muscle enzymes and how they burn fat or glucose. And I'll be talking about the fat-storing and fat-releasing enzymes found in fat cells. Like Noah, you may be thinking, "What's an enzyme?"

An enzyme is nothing more than a protein that has a fancy shape. Protein is like an iron bar. You can bend the bar and build things with it, but you can also melt it and shape it into a wrench. Then the iron would have a very specific use. Similarly, protein can be shaped for special use as an enzyme. If you don't need the wrench anymore, you can melt it down and reshape it into a screwdriver, but you still have the basic metal. Well, your body does that with protein. It can shape protein into a specific enzyme, disassemble the enzyme into its component amino acids, then put those back together as a different protein. The new protein may be another enzyme or something such as hair or skin.

Some of the enzymes we make are quite stable. Among these are the sugar-burning anaerobic enzymes in muscles. Even if you don't exercise for years, your muscles retain those enzymes because burning sugar is essential to the fight-or-flight mechanism. The fat-burning enzymes, on the other hand, break down quickly. If you don't exercise for a while, the fat-burning enzyme wrenches get rusty. We are designed so that sugar-burning enzymes last forever, but fat-burning enzymes last only if they are used. If they aren't used they break down into amino acids.

> ## "Are there enzymes I can take to increase my fat-burning ability?"

People ask, "Are there enzymes I can eat to build up my fat-burning enzymes?" And I joke that I happen to have a special sale of marathoner's "Frank Shorter" enzymes. But the truth is, *don't ever let anyone fool you into buying bottled enzymes*. Enzymes are just proteins, nothing more. The minute those enzymes hit your stomach, the acids attack them and ZAP!, their special shape is destroyed and they become ordinary proteins again.

If you don't believe me, ask a rattlesnake. Rattlesnake venom contains a special enzyme that can be lethal if it reaches the bloodstream. If you are bitten, pray for a Boy Scout to cut across the wound and suck the venom out before it gets into your blood. When I was a kid, I wondered if the Boy Scout could die from swallowing some of the poison. Not to worry! Once those enzymes hit his stomach, the acids would destroy their special shape and render them harmless.

Fat and Sugar Storage — the Gas Tanks

Each of our two fuels needs a tank. One of the tanks is pretty obvious. We know where the fat tank is because we joke about it all the time. Women store fat in certain places and men store it in others, but we have no trouble remembering where the tanks are.

Where do we store the other kind of fuel, the sugar? Are there bags of sugar scattered here and there in the body? In a sense, there are! Each muscle cell contains a little sugar and thus functions as a miniature fuel tank. When you eat candy or any food that has a lot of sugar, it becomes blood glucose, which trickles into each muscle cell. Although the amount in each cell is microscopically small, every single cell absorbs some glucose. The quadriceps, the biceps, the heart muscle, the muscles that surround the bronchial tubes — all absorb a little bit of sugar.

In the drawing on the next page, which looks a lot like the one on page 25, glucose is shown as a long chain of glucose molecules hooked together. Arranged this way, G to G to G, it is called a polymer of glucose, or glycogen. A good way to remember the word is to say out loud, "Glycogen — glucose." They sound almost the same. Or you can just call it a G-string — one that isn't going to show. In other words, in every single muscle cell in every single person there's a little G-string.

At the beginning of a run, a muscle starts using glucose by breaking off and metabolizing each molecule until it burns up

Fat and Sugar Storage

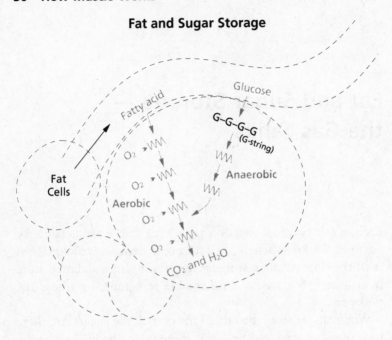

the whole G-string. The problem is that the G-string is quickly used up; the amount of energy available is quite small. So very soon the muscle sends a chemical message via the bloodstream to those tanks holding the fat. The message says, "Help! He's running! We're going to run out of G-string!" The fat cells release fatty acids, which rush to the rescue.

Fat is released from fat depots more readily in athletes than in fat people.

In athletes the fat is released from its depots more readily than it is in fat people. It's as if the fat cells in a fat person say, "Ah, heck, why hurry? He'll sit down in a minute." That's one of the reasons why the fat tanks in fat people resist getting smaller. Fat people need to exercise persistently in order to get their fat tanks to respond.

Please memorize three facts about glucose storage and three facts about fat storage:

1. Sugar is stored in the muscles.
2. It is burned first and most easily.
3. But there is very little of it so it runs out quickly.

In contrast:

1. Fat is stored far from the muscles.
2. It's a little bit harder to access when you start to exercise.
3. But it's absolutely inexhaustible.

The Krebs Cycle

On the next page is the same muscle cell diagram that I introduced earlier, but as you can see I've made it more complex. The little wiggly lines that represent enzymes are now separated into three distinct groups. Glucose and fat are not burned all the way down to carbon dioxide and water as quickly as I've suggested. They are burned down to a sort of halfway point called pyruvic acid. If you burn a white birch log and a dark oak log for a while and then put them out, they'll look much the same. The white birch isn't white anymore and the oak log doesn't look like oak. Similarly, sugar and fat look the same when half burned — they've both become pyruvic acid.

Pyruvic acid is finally metabolized to carbon dioxide and water by a third set of enzyme reactions called the Krebs cycle. Krebs was a great scientist, but most graduate students in biochemistry hate his name. Too many of us had to memorize the chemicals of the Krebs cycle with no idea why we were asked to do so. How come this guy got so famous that every chemistry student has to memorize his cycle? The Krebs cycle enzymes have some fantastic properties, one of which is the production of lots of energy — much, much, much more than is obtained from burning fat or sugar just to the pyruvate stage.

As the diagram shows, two of the enzyme groups demand oxygen, and only the group of enzymes that initiates sugar burning can operate without it. Sugar metabolism can proceed as far as pyruvic acid without oxygen, but fatty acid metabolism demands oxygen from the beginning down to pyruvic acid; then

The Krebs Cycle

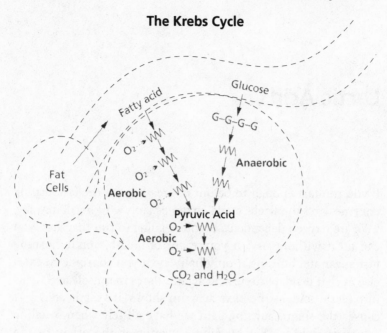

the Krebs cycle also requires oxygen to process the pyruvic acid into carbon dioxide and water.

The Krebs cycle enzymes are extremely valuable if you're playing sports that require lasting energy. When you run or play tennis, basketball, or any endurance sport, your muscles want all the energy they can get. They first grab and break apart the stored sugar molecules anaerobically, as shown in the upper right of the diagram. That provides only a little energy, so the muscles quickly direct their fat-burning enzymes (upper left) to take apart fatty acid molecules to get more energy. But it's the Krebs cycle enzymes, finishing off the metabolism of fat and sugar, that produce the bulk of the muscle's energy needs. Distance and endurance sports are impossible without the Krebs cycle.

Lactic Acid

If you run fast enough to be out of breath, both the fat-burning enzymes and the Krebs cycle enzymes stop working. They say, "We are oxygen dependent. If you're going to run that fast, you can do it without us." If you're out of breath, you're burning just sugar and burning it only halfway. If you continue to exercise at that level, pyruvic acid accumulates in muscle and turns into lactic acid, as the next diagram shows. It's lactic acid that causes the sharp, burning pain we have all felt when pedaling a bicycle uphill. That burning sensation is the origin of the expressions "Go for the burn" and "No gain without pain."

You feel the burn specifically in the muscles being used. You don't get lactic acid burn in the left leg when you exercise the right leg. Although bicycling is considered an aerobic exercise, it uses a limited amount of muscle. Work is concentrated in the quadriceps on the front of the thigh, where you feel that lactic acid burn every time you pedal up a hill. Jogging, on the other hand, involves many more muscles, including the fronts and backs of the thighs, the buttocks, the torso, and the arms. The overall effort is spread out so that no single muscle works as hard as the quadriceps during bicycling. Jogging seldom produces lactic acid except during sprinting.

By definition, the lactic acid burn means that the muscle is burning sugar halfway. Is that bad? No, it's simply a sign that the muscle is exercising AN-aerobically, burning little, if any, fat. What happens if you get the lactic acid burn during an otherwise aerobic workout? Say you're jogging comfortably but

Lactic Acid

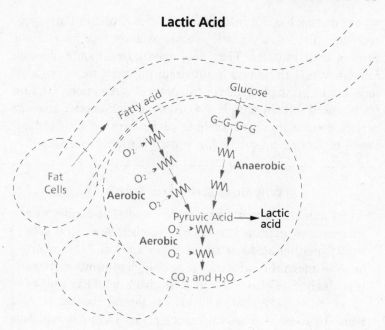

get out of breath on a short steep hill. Is your fat burning over for the day? Of course not! After you crest the hill, the lactic acid is flushed out of the muscle by the blood so that the muscle can return to aerobic metabolism. The lactic acid travels to the liver, where it is made into glucose. (Take a look at the chapter "More about Lactic Acid," page 245, for more on this.)

> **"Is your aerobic workout ruined
> if you get the lactic-acid burn?"**

Even though lactic acid production implies that no fat is being burned, sugar-burning exercise is quite beneficial in a weight-loss program because it makes muscles firm. People who lose weight through dieting alone usually jiggle a lot even after they reach a reasonable weight. They have shed pounds of fat but dieting has not made their muscles firm. Similarly, people who only do very gentle aerobic exercise lose fat without firming their muscles. They, too, may jiggle in spite of being low fat. While these people illustrate the extreme of untoned muscle, the principle applies to all of us: it is not enough to lose fat; we need to firm muscle also. Aerobic classes offer a nearly perfect combination: a half hour of fat-burning aerobics followed by lactic acid–producing, muscle-building exercises.

Why Does Lactic Acid Burn?

As its name tells you, lactic acid is acid! The acidity of a substance is indicated by its pH number. A neutral substance, neither acid nor alkaline, has a pH of 7. Numbers below 7 mean the substance is acid; higher numbers mean it is alkaline. Hydrochloric acid (stomach acid) has a pH of 2, which is *very* acid. The pH of normal muscle is 7, neutral. Severe exercise lowers the pH to 6.4 or 6.5, which may not seem like much, but it's enough to bring on a burning sensation that usually can be tolerated for only two or three minutes.

Ketosis

Let me give you another fireplace analogy. If you put a big oak log in your fireplace and light a match under it, what happens? The match goes out. What if you light a whole book of matches and hold it under the oak log? Usually nothing happens. You have to put some kindling wood under the oak log so that the match can light the kindling and the kindling can light the oak log. The Krebs cycle is like your fireplace in that the fat logs, which contain lots of calories, need sugar kindling to get them started.

I told you earlier that both fat and sugar are converted to pyruvic acid, but it's a bit more complicated than that. Fat actually burns down to a substance *like* pyruvic acid, and glucose burns down to another substance like pyruvic acid. One acts like kindling and the other like an oak log. The Krebs cycle fireplace produces most of its energy from fat logs, but unless it has some half-burned sugar molecules it has difficulty burning the fat. Sugar keeps the fire going.

> **"Do low-carbohydrate diets burn lots of fat?"**

If you looked at the diagram on page 35 without reading the text, you might think, "If I stop eating carbohydrate or sugar I'll force my muscles to burn fat only." It seems like a neat diet trick to cut out carbohydrate, forcing the muscles to burn fat exclusively, thereby speeding up fat loss. Well, it doesn't work! It doesn't work because the Krebs cycle gradually stops functioning as you run out of kindling.

Let's say you're a fat person on a low-carbohydrate diet. Pyruvic acid from fat metabolism builds up very slowly in the muscles. But because the Krebs cycle can't break down fat pyruvic acid without some sugar pyruvic acid, the pyruvic acid slowly accumulates. Instead of turning into lactic acid, it is converted to ketones. The important point is that without sugar, muscle turns fatty acids into ketones, which spill into your blood, creating a condition called ketoacidosis or ketosis. This can be measured by taking a sample of blood or urine. Some famous books that push a low-carbohydrate diet urge people to test for ketosis by dipping litmus paper in their urine. The authors claim ketosis indicates that the muscles are burning lots of fat. They're wrong. All it shows is that the muscles are burning fat *halfway*. You're not burning lots of fat, you're burning a little fat incompletely.

Emaciated Runners

Another phenomenon related to the Krebs cycle shows up in some older men who are addicted to running. You may have seen some older runners who look emaciated, especially in the upper body. Running for an hour or more every day, they use up most of the glucose kindling in the muscle cells. After the run, the muscles do everything possible to restore that glycogen and rebuild the necessary kindling supply before the next run. They snatch up any carbohydrate the runner eats and make it into stored sugar, saying, "I hope this guy doesn't go for another run before we get done."

> **Older men who are addicted to running sometimes look emaciated, especially in the upper body.**

But some dedicated runners don't give their muscles enough time. After they use up most of their stored glycogen with a morning run, the muscles try to restore it during the day. And then, before the glycogen is completely restored, they go for an afternoon run, reducing their glycogen further. At night the muscles try again to rebuild glycogen, but before it's completely rebuilt, the runner is off for a morning run again. After a while the glycogen supply decreases to the point that it's marginal

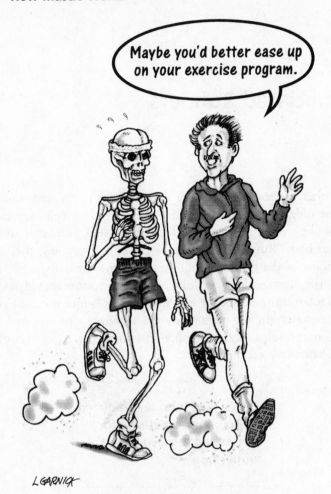

every time the runner goes for a run. When this happens the Krebs cycle is threatened because the muscle isn't getting the sugar that keeps the Krebs cycle going.

You may be confused at this point because I've repeatedly told you that fat is the primary fuel. Don't these runners use mostly fat? They do. In fact, 80 percent of their energy is coming from fat; even though they run for more than an hour, day after day, they never run out of the primary fuel. There is always fat someplace in the body. What happens is that the sugar doesn't run out in half an hour or in a day; it happens over three or four days. Eventually the muscle picks up the telephone, calls the liver, and says, "Have you got any more of that glucose stuff? We're running out down here."

The liver says, "No, we sent you the last glucose this guy ate." The muscle calls again and again until finally the liver says, "I don't have any glucose on hand, but I can take some amino acids from here and there and remove their nitrogen. Then I'll have something that looks like a glucose molecule." The liver sends a substitute kindling to the muscles to keep the Krebs cycle going. The problem is that the liver uses amino acids that were destined for some other function, primarily protein construction. The body *acts as if* it is lacking in protein no matter how much protein is in the diet. Somewhere in the body a protein-dependent tissue is going to suffer. The areas affected first are the muscles not being used. In older runners these are the neck, chest, shoulder, and arm muscles. Older men who run long distances day after day have fabulous lower-body muscles, but their upper bodies look emaciated. Now you know why.

Fat People Are Sugar Burners

The enzymes in muscle that burn glucose are emergency enzymes, designed to be retained even if we don't use them. Even if we're bedridden for weeks, we don't lose our stable sugar-burning enzymes. In contrast, we lose the fat-burning enzymes very quickly. In fact, that's almost the essence of getting "out of shape." Muscles lose their ability to burn fat, the primary fuel.

If you've gotten fat by overeating and not exercising over the last five to ten years, your muscles now can't burn the primary fuel very well. They don't know how to handle the fat anymore. When you go for a walk, your muscles burn glucose, which isn't very efficient because you run out of it quickly. Fat isn't easily lost because the muscles have forgotten how to burn it. Don't despair if you're fat. Later on I'll show you how to retrain your muscles to burn fat.

As you sit in a chair reading this book, your muscles are idling, waiting for you to get up and move — just like a car idling at a traffic light. At rest, not moving, we burn about one calorie per minute. Big people burn more than small people, but let's use one calorie per minute as our example. Part of that calorie comes from sugar and part from fat. At rest, muscles burn about 70 percent fat and 30 percent glucose.

Pretend you get on a treadmill to do a graded exercise. As you stand on the treadmill, not moving, you're burning one calorie per minute. Then you start to walk very slowly. The treadmill progressively speeds up until you are finally running to the level of exhaustion. If we could put tubes in your muscles to determine which fuel they were burning, we would find that as the number of calories per minute increases, the percentage coming from fat decreases. The faster you go, the harder it is for muscles to burn fat. The muscles use more and more calories, but they become mostly sugar calories.

> **Fat people — PAY ATTENTION!!! Getting out of shape means that muscle loses the ability to burn fat.**

On the graph on the next page you'll see that a person going from sitting to running very fast progresses from burning one calorie per minute to burning fourteen calories per minute. I don't think it is big news that the faster you go, the more calories you burn, but a fat person might conclude she should run like crazy to burn off fat. It doesn't work. Even if she didn't have a heart attack, she wouldn't lose much fat because she doesn't burn it well! The dashed lines show that fat burning decreases as the level of exercise increases. When a fat person's muscles become anaerobic, fat burning goes down to zero. Even if she increases her speed to burn more calories, she's not burning more fat calories. She's only burning sugar calories.

Elite marathon runners burn 70–80 percent fat while running. According to some research articles, the famous marathon runner Frank Shorter can run a five-minute mile while talking conversationally. You and I would be gasping. Studies of his muscles indicate that he's burning about 80 percent fat and 20 percent glucose. Frank Shorter is running aerobically while running a mile in five minutes. Your author can also do a five-minute mile — with a Honda!

Stop for a minute and think about the implications. What happens to such an athlete after a Greek island cruise during which he gains five pounds of olive oil around his waist? When

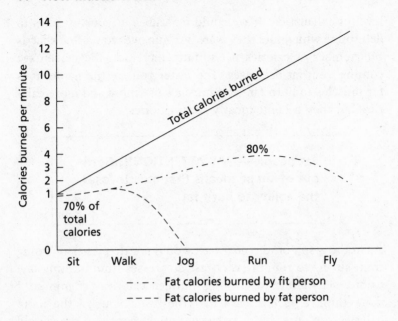

Fat calories burned by fit person
Fat calories burned by fat person

he gets home he decides to get rid of it by going for a run every day. Frank and people like him can burn twelve calories per minute, 80 percent of them fat. Roughly ten calories of fat per minute would be burned off while he runs!

Contrast that with the fat person who has brought home five pounds of extra fat from a trip to Greece and decides to run to get rid of it. If he ran fast enough to use twelve calories per minute (and he probably can't), he would burn only sugar. This person has to slow down until he reaches the point where he's still burning a significant percentage of fat. He needs to exercise as hard as he can — without getting out of breath. He needs to find the point at which he is breathing deeply but can still talk; at that point his muscles are still burning fat. For many, that level of exercise may be no more than a fast walk, at which pace he's burning three or four calories per minute. The really sad thing is that he is burning only half of those calories as fat, at most only two fat calories a minute.

Our fat person, trying his best to lose fat, can burn only two calories of fat per minute, while our super-fit person can exercise off as many as ten calories of fat per minute. As he exercises he can burn five times as much fat as his unfit friend.

If you're planning to get fat, get fit first.

The Exercise Flush

After thirty minutes of exercise, a sudden flush of fatty acids appears in the blood. Hearing that, some people conclude that we don't burn fat in our muscle until we've been exercising for thirty minutes. That is incorrect. Fatty acids are released from fat cells in a continual trickle and are burned constantly in muscle in small amounts whether you are sitting, sleeping, standing, or walking. But the minute you start exercising, muscles send signals to the fat depots, saying, "We need more than a trickle down here. *Release the grease!*" Since the fat cells are already releasing fatty acids, they don't pay much attention to the signals at first. After twenty or thirty minutes, however, they say, "All right, already! Stop badgering!" and release a gusher of fatty acids. The fatty acid level in the bloodstream suddenly rises to meet the demand. Fat is burned throughout an aerobic exercise session, even though fat cells don't release the gusher right away. The sudden peak doesn't mean that muscles are just beginning to burn fat.

> **Twenty minutes into exercise, muscles telephone the left hip, *"Release the grease!!"***

This flush of fatty acids occurs sooner in very fit athletes. Let's compare the levels of fatty acids in the blood of three individuals: an Olympic athlete, a moderately athletic person, and a couch potato. The Olympic athlete releases fatty acids before she even begins to run. Her fat cells seem to say, "She's going to run! We've got to release fatty acids right now before she starts!" The moderately athletic person might not release fatty acids for fifteen minutes, while the couch potato might not release them for thirty minutes or, if he hasn't exercised for a very long time, not at all.

The unfit person burns fat at the trickle level only; the fatty acid flush never occurs. It's almost as if his fat cells know that his muscles can't burn a lot of fatty acids, so why bother releasing them?

A very fit person whose muscles burn fatty acids well uses the sudden release almost like a fuel injection. It's a tremendous advantage to get fat released from fat cells very early in the game. In an unfit person, the early release of fatty acids wouldn't help because his muscles don't know how to burn those quantities.

3

Metabolism

People often say, "My metabolism is slowing down." What in the world are they talking about¿¿¿

Matches

The Rush to Rebuild Glycogen
How to Fix a Broken Heart

The Glycogen Window

How Fast Is Glycogen Replaced?

What *Is* Metabolism?

How Dieting Slows You Down

Matches

We need to take a second look at where the energy for muscles comes from during exercise. You might well exclaim, "Haven't you been telling us for the last umpteen chapters that the energy comes from burning fat and glucose?" It does — and it doesn't. The energy you get from fat and glucose is actually used to make a famous molecule called adenosine triphosphate or ATP. The energy from ATP is then used to contract the muscles.

Don't wince and close the book! When you think about energy and ATP, think about those old wooden matches we all used to use in the kitchen — those wooden sticks with a blob of blue stuff on the end and a little dot of red stuff on the blue stuff. Both the blue stuff and the red stuff are phosphorus, an element with so much latent energy that it virtually explodes when scratched. The red stuff is the most explosive, so it ignites first when you scratch it on the side of the box. It bursts into a very hot flame that ignites the lower-energy blue phosphorus. The blue phosphorus, in turn, lights the wooden part of the match.

Pretend that you struck such a match but immediately plunged it into water to put it out. Pretend that only the red phosphorus burned off the end, leaving the blue phosphorus and the wooden part intact. In theory you could send the match back to the factory to have the red stuff put on again. In that case you could use the match over and over. And in fact that's how muscles work. Each muscle cell has a store of ATP-matches. They are long, sticklike molecules (adenosine) with some low-energy phosphorus tipped with high-energy phosphorus. The high-energy phosphorus loves to jump off, giving you a little jolt of energy, but also doesn't mind being put back on. And luckily, muscle cells can do that. That's where fat and sugar metabolism comes in. The energy to put the phosphorus back on comes from the burning of sugar and fat.

Now you can see why I say it's sort of true and sort of not true that our muscles use sugar and fat for energy during exercise. Sugar and fat are burned, but the energy released is used to make ATP-matches.

> **Muscles burn fat and sugar,
> but it's ATP-matches that really
> make them move.**

ATP-matches are produced and used in every cell in the entire body. Even making saliva requires ATP; to take fluids out of the body and produce spit, the salivary glands need energy. Whether you're making more hair, more fingernails, new skin, or even a whole new person during pregnancy, you need lots of ATP. When a mother is breast-feeding her baby, the breast cells must convert vitamins, protein, and fluids from her blood into milk. That takes lots of energy, so breast cells use lots of ATP. Producing breast milk demands even more ATP than pregnancy.

Even the neurons in your brain transmitting electrical messages as you read and think about this book demand ATP-matches to do their job. Every cell of your entire body makes ATP-matches, uses them, and then makes them over again.

The problem with ATP-matches is that each cell has a limited supply. For most tissues this is not a problem, but what about muscle, which needs a one hundredfold increase in energy in a matter of seconds? We wouldn't be able to play much tennis if we had to rely on the ATP already in the muscle.

That's why sugar and fat burning are so important. That energy is used to reestablish the ATP-matchstick. When you use your muscles in any way, the little triphosphates on the end of the ATP molecules jump off the end, giving you a spark of energy. Then you burn a little bit of sugar or fat to produce energy to put the phosphorus back on the end of the ATP molecule and make it ready for use again. It's a complex system, but it works very, very well.

The trick is to get the ATP molecules rebuilt fast enough to keep up with the demand for energy. If you're jogging along slowly and comfortably, the ATP-matches can be used over and over. The gentle pace allows the metabolism of both sugar and fat to proceed fast enough to rebuild the ATP molecules as you use them. On the other hand, if you're sprinting, your muscles can't release energy fast enough to rebuild the ATP. The ATP-matches dwindle, and finally you have to stop running. The whole issue about energy in muscle, then, is to produce ATP fast enough to keep doing the exercise.

The Rush to Rebuild Glycogen

Exercise decreases the amount of glycogen stored in muscle. After exercise, muscles try to rebuild that glycogen as soon as possible. It's as if the muscle says, "Are you planning to exercise again in the next few minutes?" The body insists on rebuilding glycogen because of the fight-or-flight mechanism, which prepares us to defend against danger. This emergency response system, also known as the adrenaline response, depends entirely on glycogen in the muscle. Any glucose molecules available in the bloodstream are grabbed by the muscles and hooked together into G-string as fast as possible.

The muscle cell has two problems in replenishing its glycogen. First, the glucose has to get into the muscle. A muscle cell membrane has little pores in it that allow vitamins, fluids, and such to trickle in and out. But those pores are a little bit tight for glucose molecules. To facilitate their entry, insulin makes those little holes dilate, almost the way your pupil dilates in the dark. After a sugary meal, insulin, secreted from the pancreas, travels in blood to all the muscles saying, "Open up, baby, let the Ding-Dong in."

After exercise, muscle, eager to have its glucose, reacts almost as if it's in an emergency situation. When you eat sugar, your insulin level rises quickly and the muscle absorbs the sugar quickly. So sugar, if it's available, enters muscle cells more readily after exercise.

The second problem is to make that glucose into glycogen. Any time you hook one molecule of sugar to another, it takes a bit of energy. Where's your muscle going to get the energy to make those chemical bonds? ATP, right? Some of the ATP in the muscle cell comes rushing up, splits off its red-hot phosphorus, and liberates the energy needed to cement one glucose molecule to another.

Sounds easy enough — but what happens after a long hard exercise, when I've used up all my ATP? Now I'm driving home after my run with sugar in my blood from a Ding-Dong. Insulin comes to my muscle and opens the door for the sugar, but there's no ATP in there. How is the muscle cell going to make glycogen? Fat to the rescue! Remember, as I've said over and over, fat molecules are abundant. We may run out of sugar, but we never run out of fat. As I'm driving, fatty acid molecules are slowly taken apart by enzymes and their energy used to re-manufacture ATP-matches. The ATP-matches are then used to cement the glucose molecules together. In other words, we burn fat after an exercise to get the energy to synthesize glycogen. We break down fat in order to build up glycogen.

> **"If fat is burned only during aerobic exercise, why aren't sprinters fat?"**

Sometimes I challenge my audiences with the question, "Why aren't sprinters fat?" If the only time we burn fat is when we're exercising aerobically, then sprinters, weightlifters, and anyone who does stop-and-go sports should be fat. But you can see now that a sprinter, while she's sitting on the edge of the track after a sprint, is metabolizing fat in order to make ATP in order to resynthesize glycogen for her next sprint. Because of the intensity of the workout, a sprinter's aerobic system is "revved up" during recovery. The reason sprinters aren't fat is that they burn a lot of fat during their recovery from sprinting. They don't burn fat when they sprint, but they burn lots of it when they rest after the exercise. Similarly, you don't burn fat when you weightlift; you burn it only afterward when the muscles are recovering.

ALL athletes are low in fat because they ALL burn lots of fat during recovery, but the reason I emphasize low-intensity aerobic exercise such as bicycling or fast walking for my fat readers is that they get the benefit of fat burning both during and after exercise. You always burn fat AFTER exercise, but you burn fat DURING exercise only if it's aerobic.

How to Fix a Broken Heart

The heart is just a specialized muscle, which contracts like a biceps and metabolizes fatty acids like a calf muscle — and — and — and — it depends on glycogen like any other muscle. After hard, prolonged exercise, the heart, too, must replace glycogen to prepare for fight or flight. Something tells me it is more vital to get my heart ready for an emergency than my gluteus maximus. Wouldn't it be neat if the sugar from the candy I eat after exercise could be preferentially directed to rebuild heart glycogen? Believe it or not, we have a built-in mechanism that allows that to happen. The heart synthesizes all the glycogen it needs BEFORE glucose is made available to leg, buttocks, arm, or any other muscle. Even though the blood is carrying glucose through all the other glycogen-starved muscles, they don't get a drop until the heart is satisfied. The heart replaces its glycogen first, then the major muscles fill up, and finally, after all the others have eaten their fill, if any sugar is left in the blood, the liver's storehouse begins to refill.

We don't yet understand the mechanism that gives the heart its preferential status. We also don't know why the liver so politely waits its turn while the skeletal muscles eat all they want. Just when we think we are starting to understand how the human body works, something like this mystery of the heart makes us humble again.

The Glycogen Window

After long, intense exercise, the muscles scream, "Emergency! Emergency!" and do everything they can to rebuild glycogen. Eating pure junk-food sugar is the best way to speed up the process. Before you clap, saying, "Whoopee! Ding-Dongs from now on!" you need to know that this solution doesn't apply after a mere twenty- to forty-minute aerobic workout. It's only for athletes who exercise hard and long enough to significantly deplete their glycogen.

The "glycogen window" refers to the two hours immediately following such hard exercise. During those two hours eating ordinary table sugar will raise the level of glycogen in your muscles faster than anything else. I realize this flies in the face of all the rules nutritionists are trying to teach us. We are told to eat complex carbohydrates like breads, cereals, and pasta and to avoid sugary junk food. But those admonishments to avoid sugar are coming from research on fat people, not fit athletes. If we asked our fit athletes what they need to get pepped up again after intense exercise, they'd probably say, "Sugar." For about two hours after an intense workout they eat candy, Jell-O, sugary drinks — anything with a very high sugar content.

After the two-hour orgy, however, sugar offers no further advantage. It's better to shift to the long-chain carbohydrates that we are more typically encouraged to eat.

Glycogen is replaced up to 50 percent faster in athletes who eat immediately than in those who wait a couple of hours. The muscles say, "Hey! we want to make glycogen *now*, not two hours from now."

A lot of athletes can't stomach solid food after exercise, so they rely on sugary drinks. Fruit juices provide liquid carbohydrate, but the fructose in them isn't absorbed as readily as glucose. You'll probably get a faster rate of glycogen synthesis by drinking one of the commercial "after exercise" drinks such as Gatorlode, Carboplex, or Exceed High Carbohydrate Source. (Take a look at the chapter "Sports Drinks" for more on glucose absorption.)

> **The fastest way to replace glycogen after intense exercise is to eat pure junk-food sugar.**

Restoring glycogen requires a lot of energy, which burns lots of calories, which in turn produces lots of heat. That's where most of the heat comes from that athletes experience after an exercise. Most people assume that the heat is "left over," residual from the exercise itself, much the way a car engine stays hot after it's been running for a while. But the heat of exercise is dissipated in minutes because of the incredible efficiency of our heat-releasing systems. The heat you feel an hour or more after exercise is predominantly the heat of glycogen resynthesis. It's the same as saying your metabolism is elevated.

Fat people trying to diet away their pounds complain about having a slow metabolism. They don't exercise intensely, so their bodies have no need to replace glycogen. Of course their metabolism is down! And as if that weren't bad enough, when they eat a sweet dessert, it doesn't end up as muscle glycogen for tomorrow's exercise; it's converted into triglyceride and dumped into fat cells.

How Fast Is Glycogen Replaced?

After all this talk about the body's need to replace glycogen, we should look at some numbers. How fast does glycogen go back into the muscle after hard, long exercise? In the average person, muscle glycogen is replaced at a rate of approximately 5 percent per hour. The muscles of extremely fit athletes can absorb up to 10 percent per hour.

Let's talk first about Average Joe, who replaces glycogen at the rate of 5 percent an hour. Suppose he goes for a five-day hike, backpacking with a heavy pack. He gradually loses glycogen as he hikes. Even though his muscles are using fat as the predominant fuel, they still need a little bit of glycogen kindling for every step he takes. The fat fuel is not going to run out, but the glycogen may. As he walks along the trail, he uses more glycogen than he is able to replace even if he's eating as he hikes.

Let's say he hikes for three or four hours and decreases his stored glycogen by 40 percent. Then he stops beside the trail for a huge meal. I don't care how much he eats or what he eats, even pure table sugar, it is only going to go back into the muscles at the rate of 5 percent per hour. If his glycogen is decreased by 40 percent it's going to take eight hours to put it back in again. After the meal, he starts hiking again. The carbohydrate from the meal slowly goes to his muscles, replenishing glycogen. The problem is that even if the glycogen is going into his muscles at the rate of 5 percent per hour, his hiking may be depleting it at 15 percent per hour. Only at night when he falls into his sleeping bag does glycogen get replenished without being tapped. However, at 5 percent per hour there's a good chance that by the next morning he won't be back up to 100 percent glycogen again. He may start the day with only 95 percent glycogen, which decreases all day long. By the fifth day he'll run out of kindling. As described in the chapter "Emaciated Runners," that's the point at which protein starts to be used as fuel.

> **"How come skinny, fit runts can hike longer than big, strong macho types?"**

The beauty of exercise is that our muscles can be trained to store more glycogen. Muscle adapts to the constant demand for replacement glycogen by allowing sugar to enter the cell more quickly. This is caused by an increase in muscle sensitivity to insulin. It takes less insulin to get the sugar to enter the cell. (Obviously, this has ramifications if you have diabetes in your family or any other insulin problem.)

Elite athletes can replace as much as 10 percent of their glycogen per hour. These are the people whose glycogen won't be gone at the end of a four-day hike. Skinny little runners just keep hiking day after day, still burning glycogen long after Average Joe's exhausted muscles have switched to protein for fuel.

What *Is* Metabolism?

People talk about metabolism as if it were a simple thing. They use the word so readily and so frequently, you would think that its meaning was quite clear. But if you look up "metabolism" in a textbook of medicine, you'll find hundreds of pages on the subject. Medical students spend an entire semester studying carbohydrate metabolism. Just when they start thinking they're hotshot metabolic wizards, their professors throw a semester of fat metabolism at them. That's followed by protein metabolism and liver metabolism, and on and on.

Why is it that a word that seems perfectly understandable to most of us requires years of study by the medical profession? It must have a deeper, more complex meaning beyond the layman's definition. Basically, metabolism is ALL the chemical reactions that occur in your body, all the reactions that take place in your brain, liver, digestive tract, muscles, heart, lungs, and every other tissue or organ. You can see that a thorough understanding of metabolism would require years of study.

I hope my medical friends will forgive me, but let's face it, the public equates metabolism with calorie burning. After all, the fat guy on the street isn't thinking about all those chemical reactions when he says, "I've gained twenty pounds and I'm not eating any more than before. My metabolism must be slowing down." All he knows is that he's gaining weight on less food.

When your mother says, "You know, dear, your metabolism slows down as you get older," she's not thinking about compli-

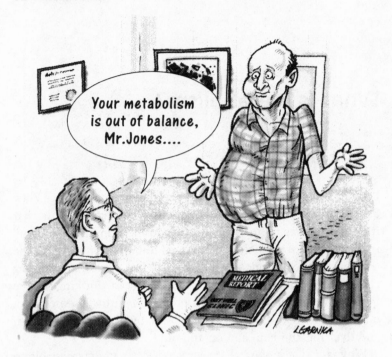

Your metabolism is out of balance, Mr. Jones....

cated physiology. She just knows that you don't burn as many calories when you're older.

Physicians and dietitians have only themselves to blame for the public's easy use of their complex word, for they, too, explain away weight gain or loss by saying, "Your metabolism is changing." If I seem to be able to eat lots of calories without gaining weight, they say I have a fast metabolism. If I gain weight on a leaf of lettuce, they say my metabolism is slow.

So — for the sake of this chapter, when I talk about metabolism, I'll simply be referring to calorie burning. How many do you use and how do you use them?

Basal metabolic rate (BMR) is the number of calories the body uses just to exist, to lie in bed and breathe. Unfortunately, BMR is not a very useful tool because it's difficult to measure. The person being tested is put into unfamiliar surroundings, attached to some wires, and told to go to sleep. Even if he can sleep under such bizarre circumstances, he'll probably have high-energy nightmares. The impracticality of BMR has generated a more useful measurement called resting metabolic rate (RMR). The person is asked to rest in a comfortable chair, relax as much as possible, and simulate the energy level of reading a book.

As you sit reading this book, you are probably metabolizing slightly more calories than if you were sound asleep. If you are a woman, your BMR might be 800 and your RMR about 100 calories above that. A large woman's basal metabolism may be higher than 800, and a smaller woman's BMR may be lower. And RMR may be 150 calories more or only 50 calories. In any case, the increase in calories from BMR to RMR is small.

"How come I'm getting fatter on the same amount of food?"

On the graph on the next page you can see the additive effect of all the facets of metabolism and the approximate number of calories for each. The graph is for an average woman — men, please extrapolate. BMR is shown at the bottom of the bar; notice that it represents more than half the bar. Even if our average woman were in a coma, she would need about 800 calories. Assuming she is not in a coma but living a normal life, we can add 100 calories for her resting metabolic rate, raising her total to 900.

Some people fidget when you ask them to relax. They never stop moving. They scratch, they look up and look around, they cross and recross their legs; in short, they don't really sit still. It's hard to determine their resting metabolic rate because they don't rest. For such people (often called teenagers), we add a new metabolism category, called fidget, to the graph. At this point our average woman is metabolizing about 1,000 calories a day:

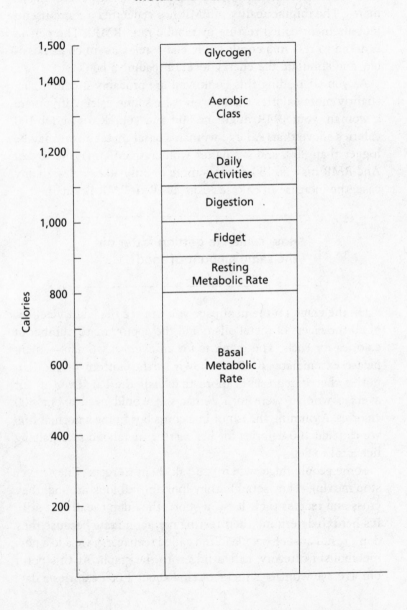

An Average Woman's Metabolism and Calories Used

800 for BMR, 100 more to read a book, and 100 more because she's hyper.

Let's add still another category to the metabolism of our average woman — digestion. You may have noticed that after eating a large meal you tend to feel hot. You may even perspire. This heat comes from digesting your food. After eating, our average woman's liver, pancreas, stomach, and intestines have to produce digestive enzymes. This uses up calories at the same time that digestion produces calories from food. There is a dilemma here. If our average woman is gaining weight and feels that her metabolism is slowing down, she may decide to eat less, which means she will digest less, which depresses her metabolism even further.

Never mind how many calories are in the food. The point is, digestion contributes to metabolism. The more she eats, and the more often she eats, the more her digestive organs have to gear up to handle the food. On our graph I've added 100 calories for average digestion.

Our average woman also has normal daily activities such as showering, getting dressed, driving a car, shopping, and walking around her office. I'm not talking about planned exercise sessions, but rather the activities of everyday life. For this category I have added another 100 calories to her day's metabolism, labeled daily activity.

We now have a grand total of 1,200 calories. This is the maintenance number most often prescribed by qualified nutritionists. It assumes that the average, healthy, normal woman needs about 1,200 calories each day to maintain her weight.

Let's send our average woman to aerobic class three times a week. She burns 9 calories per minute during her sixty minutes of exercise. Spread out over a week, this comes to about 250 calories a day, which I have added to the graph in the category of aerobic class.

Finally we have to consider what happens *after* exercise. People get so hung up on the number of calories used during exercise that they forget about all the calorie-burning processes that happen afterward. Glycogen has to be replaced in the muscles, triglycerides in the fat cells need to be restored. The harder and more prolonged the exercise, the greater the demand for fuel replenishment afterward. I have labeled the category covering all the metabolic events necessary after mild exercise simply glycogen.

Plenty of women who think of themselves as normal and healthy maintain their weight on 900 calories a day. They have no obvious malfunction or overt sickness. They complain of a depressed metabolism, imagining their basal metabolic rate to be at fault. In fact their BMR may be steady at 800 calories per day, just as when they were younger and able to eat like crazy without gaining weight. Their decreased metabolism can be explained by examining the other metabolic categories.

> **"Is it true that exercise speeds up metabolism?"**

If they don't go to an aerobic class or similar planned exercise, their need for glycogen decreases. They may also unconsciously slow down in other ways so that their daily-activities metabolism is depressed. They eat less and therefore digest less. They can read or have a conversation without fidgeting, which further reduces total metabolism. They don't keep warm through movement so they wear sweaters and turn up the heat, and their internal heat production may go down. All of these changes are reversed if they get into a regular exercise program.

You can see now why no one has made sense out of metabolism before. It is made up of many little metabolisms, any one of which can change without showing any change in the BMR tested at a clinic. If you are getting fat with no change in the number of calories you're eating, you must wonder which one of all those calorie-demanding processes has changed. We say metabolism is slowing down as if it were a single process or a single switch that controls one process. But thousands of metabolic processes are happening every minute of every day. Certainly they don't ALL slow down at once. Can you pinpoint which metabolic process has changed to make you fat? No! You can't, and your physician can't, and your mother can't. But it doesn't matter, because almost all of them can be increased if you add exercise to your life. Don't focus on the number of calories burned _during_ exercise — think about the metabolic consequences of exercise.

How Dieting Slows You Down

Think of all the metabolic processes that work hard to replace glycogen after exercise. The liver snatches carbohydrates from your last meal, makes them into glucose, and packs them off to the muscles. The liver also converts amino acids into glucose. The pancreas works hard after exercise to make insulin so that sugar can enter the muscles. Then there is the obvious demand for energy when sugar is made into glycogen in the muscle itself. Finally, fatty acids are burned in the muscle to produce the energy to synthesize glycogen.

Where do fatty acids come from? They come from fat cells, don't they? Fat cells throughout the body are releasing — metabolizing — fatty acids, and that process requires energy. In the muscle, energy is needed to burn the fat molecules in order to make energy to make the glycogen. Talk about complex! Even lactic acid gets into the act. The liver says, "Oh, brother! Here's some lactic acid. What am I supposed to do with it?" The liver puts the lactic acid through chemical changes, makes it into sugar, and sends it back to the muscle, where it can be made into glycogen.

A lot of metabolism takes place in the body after exercise. Most people think they've stopped using calories, but they haven't. All of these metabolic processes work madly to accomplish just one goal — to replace muscle glycogen — which is just one of the metabolism categories in the graph on page 64. With such an enormous impact in this one category, imagine the effect exercise has on all the other categories!

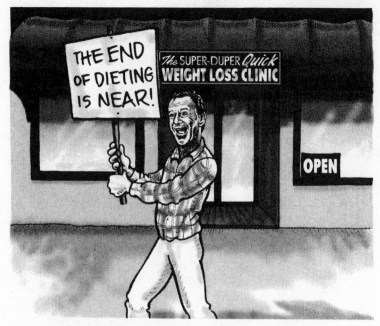

Bailey continues his crusade....

Overweight people sign up for expensive diet programs because their metabolism is slow. Even responsible physicians prescribe diet programs that only treat fat people's symptoms, doing nothing to "fix" their metabolism. The most popular diet programs are the ones that make people lose weight fast, which depresses their metabolism even further. Instead of helping people speed up their slow metabolism, these programs make the problem worse.

None of the weight-loss diets increases even one of the glycogen-building processes. Exercise enhances all of them.

4

Exercise Basics

*This section is a "how to" that will rescue you
from all the "how to" books.*

Aerobic Exercise Equals Systemic Exercise

Don't Depend on Heart Rate

Your Exercise Speedometer

A "Set Point" for Fitness

How Hard Should I Exercise?

The Aerobic Zone

How Often Should I Exercise?

Overtraining

How to Avoid Overtraining

How to Get Fit Fast

Bicycling versus Cross-Country Skiing

Cross Training

Natural Exercise versus Machines

Aerobic Exercise Equals Systemic Exercise

When evaluating an exercise, ask if it affects one part of the body or the whole body. If you had an infected cut on your finger, a doctor would say you had a local infection. If the infection spread to the rest of your body, he would call it a systemic infection. Jogging appears to be just a local leg exercise, but it affects your lungs, liver, heart, and bones, qualifying it as a systemic exercise. In contrast, weightlifting affects the muscles used but has relatively little effect on the rest of the body.

The focus of this book is on endurance, total-body exercises that induce systemic changes and improve health. Doctors recommend my books because I talk about the systemic benefits of exercise, not about exercise making bigger biceps.

The term "aerobic exercise" was invented to describe *systemic* exercise. When the term was first used, the press made it seem like a startling new discovery, but doctors have known for a long time that certain kinds of exercise improve the health of the whole body. In practical terms any exercise is aerobic if it

1. Lasts at least twelve minutes without stopping.
2. Gets you breathing deeply but not out of breath.
3. And uses the muscles in the thighs and buttocks.

Exercise that fulfills these three criteria elicits systemic changes. Aerobic or systemic — the words can be used interchangeably.

> **Doctors recommend exercise for its systemic benefits, not because it makes bigger biceps.**

Don't Depend on Heart Rate

Athletes running their fastest can almost always squeeze out a little extra speed for a few seconds. Perhaps their lungs open a little more or their muscles contract a little faster. Somewhere, some organ contributes a little more than its "maximum." But not the heart; it stubbornly levels out at its maximum pumping speed. Of course, that maximum is different for each person, but for an individual the maximum is quite consistent regardless of the type of exercise, the time, or even the altitude. If an individual goes from being extremely out of shape to being very fit, there is no change in maximum heart rate. The only factor that does affect it is age; maximum heart rate decreases inexorably as we get older.

The heart is a muscle that contracts and relaxes all day long. Age doesn't change its speed of contraction, but it does change the speed of relaxing. Try squashing a worn-out tennis ball in one hand. Use a flimsy one that doesn't require much muscle strength. Squash the ball, then relax and squash it again repeatedly as fast as you can. If this were shown in slow motion, you would see that an older person squashes the ball as fast as a young person, but it takes the older person longer to open his hand for the next squeeze. In other words, relaxing a muscle takes longer as we get older. The heart, being a muscle, takes longer to prepare itself for the next contraction.

Knowing this about the heart, researchers devised a formula for how much heart rate decreases with age. By having people of all ages run at their maximum on a treadmill, they came up with a general formula: 220 minus your age equals maximum heart rate: $220 - \text{age} = \text{MHR}$. Unfortunately, this formula is only an average; 30 to 40 percent of us don't fit the formula because our hearts go slower or faster than the age-predicted maximum. The only way to know your maximum heart rate accurately is to be tested at maximum, as in the oxygen uptake test described in Part One. But a maximum treadmill test is expensive and, as pointed out before, it's hard on the person being tested, even carrying the risk of heart attack. I don't recommend it except in special circumstances.

You can do your own maximum test simply by exercising to exhaustion and having someone take your pulse. This should be quite accurate, since taking a six-second pulse doesn't require a lot of skill. I have taken my own many times while on cross-country skis. While skiing uphill slowly, but carrying a day pack and wearing lots of winter clothing, I can easily exercise right up to my maximum. Because I'm going slowly, I can take my pulse at the same time. Here again, however, testing yourself carries some degree of risk. While attempting a basically simple test, you could have a heart attack, which sort of defeats the point.

> **The exercise heart rate charts on gym walls aren't as reliable as people think.**

I'm *not* saying everyone should take his or her own maximum heart rate. Finding your own maximum is a personal decision, just like the decision to do maximum-intensity sports. Without knowing a lot more about you, I can't advise you to do it.

It would simplify discussions about exercise if we all knew our real, honest-to-goodness maximum heart rate. But many of us don't. All the charts for heart-monitored exercise, even the ones in my original *Fit or Fat?* depend on the 220 − age formula. These charts are so popular that people who don't fit the formula use them anyway, with the result that they may not be exercising in their true aerobic range.

Suppose, for example, you are cross-country skiing, jogging, walking, or bicycling at a familiar, comfortable pace. You stop, take a six-second pulse, and multiply by ten to get the number of heartbeats per minute. Wow! your heart rate is much higher (or lower) than it's supposed to be! — according to the heart rate charts. Don't panic. You're not sick or weird or exercising incorrectly. You are just like me and one-third of the rest of the population. Our hearts don't fit the 220 − age = MHR formula. We have to use common sense when we exercise rather than depend on somebody else's numbers.

If you don't know your true maximum heart rate, you're probably better off if you throw those charts away. I have a Home Fitness Test on page 175 that doesn't use heart rate at all. Instead, you rely on breathing and comfort level to determine the intensity of your exercise. If you're breathing comfortably and talking easily during exercise, you're probably below the aerobic level. If you're breathing deeply but not gasping, talking haltingly but not gabbing, you're exercising aerobically. If you're wheezing and unable to string more than three words together, you're above the level of aerobic exercise and into the anaerobic level.

Your Exercise Speedometer

I have a new way of splitting exercise into various levels of intensity. I call it my exercise "speedometer."

The activity zones on my speedometer are not exact. You'll know when you are solidly in the middle of a zone, but at the transitions they blend together — like the colors of a rainbow. It's easy to identify the middle of the orange band, but it is hard to pinpoint exactly where orange changes to red on one side or to yellow on the other.

Rest and recuperation occur when the heart beats at less than 50 percent of its maximum. This is the time when muscle glycogen is replaced, aerobic enzymes are built, and muscle growth takes place. It does no good to design the perfect weight-lifting, wind-sprinting, or aerobic exercise program if recuperation is not included. You can exercise all you want, but if you don't give your muscles rest, your fitness won't improve. Fit people have resting heart rates as low as 25 percent of maximum (40–50 beats per minute), which gives them a very wide zone in which to recuperate. The resting heart rate of fat, out-of-shape people is often as high as 45 percent of maximum (75–90 beats per minute), so their recuperation zone is very narrow.

Very fit people have two advantages when they rest. First, their wide recuperation zone enables them to handle physical or emotional stress better. When a fit person gets the flu, for example, his heart rate may increase up to 35 percent of maximum, but he is still in his recuperation zone. When an unfit

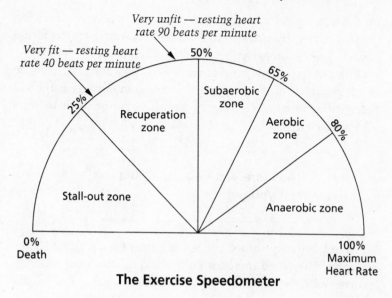

The Exercise Speedometer

person gets the flu his heart rate pushes him out of the recuperation zone so tissue repair is jeopardized.

Second, very fit people can be active and still be in their recuperation zone. When fit teenage Johnny gets a cold, his mom wants him to rest. For her, rest means sitting down. For Johnny, playing Frisbee or shooting hoops with his friends in the driveway may be rest. It takes a lot of running around to drive him above 50 percent maximum heart rate. Fit people rest and recuperate while having fun doing active things.

Don't overlook the significance of this: it may be the most important thing you'll ever learn about fitness. Fat, out-of-shape people often complain of how hard it is to get fit again. They try to exercise religiously, but something always seems to go wrong, causing repeated setbacks. Their recuperation zone is so narrow that it's hard to stay within it. Even if they exercise perfectly, monitoring their breathing and heart rate, the slightest cold, muscle strain, or stress drives them above that narrow zone, thus decreasing the time spent in recuperation. Fit people, on the other hand, appear not to need rest. When they're doing gentle activity, they're still in their recuperation zone, repairing tissue, replenishing glycogen, and building muscle.

Out-of-shape people need to exercise gently and rest, exercise gently and rest, over and over until they gradually get fitter and their resting heart rate gradually decreases, giving them an ever-widening zone in which to recuperate.

> **The more you sit around, the less rest you get.**

I have arbitrarily named the 50–65 percent range the subaerobic zone. This zone includes golf, walking, and your author's favorite pastime, mountain hiking. When I hike, I'm in the subaerobic zone most of the time. Occasional uphills push me into the aerobic zone, and very steep climbs push me into the anaerobic zone. But most of the time I just amble along subaerobically, enjoying the scenery. Because I do so much of it, I'm quite sure my subaerobic pastime does more to maintain my fitness than the aerobic jogging I do when I'm home. Keep this in mind when you read the chapters on walking.

Exercising with the heart rate between 65 and 80 percent of MHR is the most efficient way to produce the systemic effects that we associate with aerobic exercise. Notice the word efficient! You can get aerobic benefits from subaerobic exercise, as I do with my mountain hiking, but you have to do a lot of it. Mountain hiking works, but not efficiently. It can't be called aerobic exercise even though it yields aerobic benefits. This distinction has really confused a lot of people. Some feel that any exercise above or below the 65–80 percent MHR range is worthless. They ask, "If I'm jogging aerobically on the level and encounter an uphill that gets me out of breath, have I ruined my whole exercise because I've gone into the anaerobic zone?" Definitely not! Like my hiking, mixing subaerobic, aerobic, and anaerobic exercise yields systemic benefits. The 65–80 percent range is merely a guideline to help people pick the exercise that most *efficiently* induces systemic improvements. While both intense, anaerobic exercise and mild, low-key activity will produce spinoff systemic benefits, the closer they come to moderate aerobic exercise the faster these changes occur.

What if the exercise we do is never aerobic? Suppose we put a hundred fat men, who haven't lifted an exercise finger in a decade, on a low-intensity golf program. They have to walk eighteen holes of golf every day towing their clubs on a cart. We strap heart rate monitors around their chests to be sure they never exceed 60 percent of their maximum heart rate. Unlike my mountain hiking, which is mainly subaerobic but has bouts of aerobic and anaerobic activity, the exercise never moves them out of their subaerobic zone. But even though they're only exercising at 60 percent MHR, their results on an oxygen uptake test would improve. At the end of six months they would definitely be more fit than when they started. Conclusion: golf is an aerobic exercise? No! It's a subaerobic exercise that will produce systemic benefits in relatively unfit people if it's done enough.

Judge exercise by its effects, not by an artificial number. Too many aerobic instructors, personal trainers, and club owners are so focused on heart rate that they overlook this point. Almost any exercise can increase your oxygen uptake and improve your health. The 65–80 percent MHR exercise zone is an efficiency guide, not a dictum.

A "Set Point" for Fitness

People are familiar with the concept of "set point" when applied to weight; our bodies tend to return to a set weight in spite of our good — or bad — efforts to change it. If we diet stringently we lose weight, but once we stop dieting we bounce right back up to our original weight. Similarly, if we overindulge during the holidays, we put on some pounds, but usually we lose them when we go back to normal eating.

Now here's an intriguing idea. Is there a set point for fitness? I believe each person has a level of fitness that is easily maintained, a level the body readily returns to after periods of non-exercise that fits the concept of set point. It takes little effort to move up from a level of very low fitness to one's set point, but it takes concentrated effort to go above that to a higher level.

The concept of set point helps answer a lot of questions about how much exercise one has to do to get fit and stay fit. Most of the questions involve three variables:

- How often to exercise — frequency
- How long to exercise — duration
- How hard to exercise — intensity

On the graph the three variables are combined into one, called effort. The amount of effort people put out to be fit directly affects their oxygen uptake, that is, their fitness level. A low amount of effort yields a low level of fitness. However, notice that initially it doesn't take much effort to become *more*

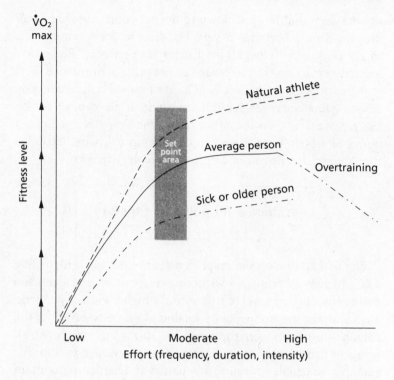

fit. Assuming they don't get hurt or suffer some other setback (as mentioned in "Your Exercise Speedometer"), people who are very unfit respond well to exercise; their fitness levels go up quite quickly. Fitness level continues to rise as the person puts more effort into exercise. But at a certain level of effort, fitness reaches a plateau or set point where it seems to resist further improvement. On my graph I show this area as a bend to the right. Beyond that point it becomes more and more difficult to raise your fitness level. Athletes have to make an enormous effort to improve. They have to exercise long, hard, and often to become a little better at their sport because they are already above their "natural" set point.

When an athletic person takes a few weeks off, her performance drops quickly. Her actual fitness level — oxygen uptake —

doesn't drop that far, just down to her set point. But that small drop in fitness becomes a very big drop in performance. She might complain, "I lost all my fitness in one week!" She *didn't* lose all her fitness, but to return to her prior performance level requires many grueling weeks of hard exercise because her body resists going above its natural set point. If an average person takes a week off, on the other hand, she drops below her set point. Her body is so eager to get back up to its natural level that she regains fitness and performance very quickly.

> ## "Is there a set point for fitness?"

The dashed line on the graph depicts the natural athlete. She has a higher set point, so without exercising a great deal, she maintains a higher level of fitness and a higher level of performance than the average person. The dotted line is reserved for the person who doesn't get the usual payoff for her efforts. At all levels of fitness, she works harder than the average person. For example, as people get older, it is harder and harder to maintain fitness. There are some very fit eighty-year-olds, but most of them admit they work a lot harder to stay that way than they did when they were young. People who have the flu or are systemically ill are in the same boat.

The graph also helps us visualize the concept of overtraining (which I explain later in "Overtraining"); although you put out more and more effort, your level of fitness actually goes down. Your mother would capture the concept with the phrase, "You're trying too hard, dear." People who overtrain are usually much more fit than their friends, so that a friend's advice to take it easy is ignored. They rationalize that their unfit friends don't understand the subtleties of training. They exercise harder and harder, assuming that their performance deterioration is just a phase.

If you accept the idea of a set point for fitness, you should now understand what seems to be contradictory exercise advice. I tell super-fit Susan to exercise long, hard, and often to get a small improvement, but couch potato Mary needs only a moderate amount of exercise to see a big improvement.

How Hard Should I Exercise?

Of the three variables of exercise — intensity, duration, and frequency — intensity drives fitness levels up most quickly. Whether you are super fit or totally out of shape, make your workout more intense if you want to improve in a hurry.

What seems like a drawback to intense exercise is that it burns sugar, not fat. A fat person, hearing that intense exercise is the best way to get fit but that it doesn't burn any fat, might say, "Why should I do it?" The answer is, if he sticks with low-intensity aerobic exercise, his body never learns to burn fat at higher levels of exercise. By including occasional intense exercise, his fat-burning potential goes up. His body learns to be aerobic at levels of exercise that once were anaerobic.

> **Exercise for getting fit is not the same as exercise for losing fat.**

Let me clarify my use of the word "intensity." Let's say you are terribly out of shape and fifty pounds overfat; slow walking is your fastest comfortable exercise. In the middle of your walk you go up a short hill, which makes you puff a little. The uphill is not hard enough or long enough to exhaust you or make you gasp, but it's enough extra effort to make you glad to reach the top. That little hill represents the level of intensity I'm talking about. Sprinting madly up the hill as if it were an emergency would be too intense for you. On the other hand, an Olympic runner might zoom up the same hill by adding relatively little effort to his comfortable run. Intensity is a relative term — it means pushing yourself above what's comfortable.

The problem with intense exercise is that it can produce more accidents. A runner pushing hard to improve is vulnerable to shin splints, tendinitis, torn or twisted ligaments, and other injuries that will prevent him from running at all. The injury defeats the purpose of doing the hard run in the first place. Because of the risk of injury, few books talk about the benefits of intensity.

I've got good news! There are three classic ways to add intensity to a program while minimizing the risk of injury: wind sprints, cross training, and weightlifting.

Wind sprints, briefly adding extra effort as in my example above, increase intensity for such short periods that you can avoid fatigue and injury.

In cross training, we ask muscles that are usually used in one way to move in a different way. Since these muscles are not used to the new exercise, the work required is more intense for them. By switching from one moderate activity to another moderate activity you can fool the muscles into thinking they're exercising more intensely.

Adding weightlifting to an aerobic program is yet another way of increasing intensity while providing protection against injury. Lifting heavy weights not only works muscles intensely, it also makes them stronger so that they protect joints and ligaments from injury. Weightlifting, especially with machines, allows you to work out very intensely with relative safety. Weightlifting is not aerobic or fat burning, but it rapidly energizes after-exercise metabolic effects.

Now the next chapter, "The Aerobic Zone," gives good reasons to avoid intense exercise, seemingly a contradiction to this chapter. Not so! Do the long, steady part of your exercise at the low end of the aerobic zone, with short periods of more intense exercise as detailed in this chapter. That way you get the best of both worlds.

The Aerobic Zone

When we talk about the aerobic zone, 65–80 percent of maximum heart rate, everybody asks, "Where in the zone should I exercise?" Or, "Should my pace be a little on the easy side or a little on the hard side?" As the last chapter showed, you'll improve most quickly by exercising at the upper end of the zone, around 80 percent. But that doesn't work for everybody. In recent years, more and more research shows that exercising at the lower level of the aerobic zone is far more beneficial than we used to think.

The advantages of lower-level exercise were first noted in older people. A study was done comparing two groups of men averaging seventy years of age. Half ran around a high school track every day at a speed that got their hearts up to 65 percent of maximum. The other half went around the track with their hearts going at about 80 percent of maximum. Both groups were tested periodically to see if they were getting fitter. Were their lungs getting better and their hearts stronger? Were the fat-burning enzymes in their muscles increasing? Surprisingly, the researchers found that the men who exercised at 65 percent showed more improvement than the men who exercised at 80 percent. The reason is that at age seventy, your body doesn't repair itself as fast as it did when you were twenty. When the men who exercised at 80 percent rested, their bodies said, "Do you want us to grow enzymes or repair tissue? We can't do both." They needed to rest more or to exercise at a lower level.

Just as age restricts us because we synthesize proteins less

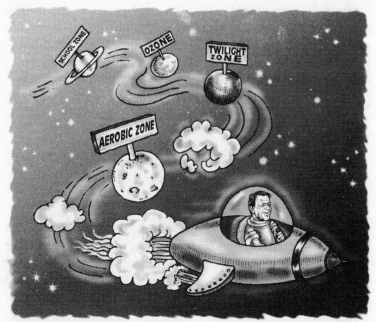

L GARNICA

quickly and less well, illness is also a restriction. Suppose you have a cold that makes you feel a little debilitated, but not enough to stop you from doing your usual exercise. If you exercise at 80 percent of your maximum heart rate, that night your body will say, "I can't fight this infection and build muscle at the same time." Even if you are thirty years old, your body will respond as if you were one of those seventy-year-old men.

A bad diet, either extremely unbalanced or very low in calories, can also pose a significant threat to the building of tissue. If you're one of those zealots eating 800 calories or less and exercising every day at 80 percent of maximum heart rate, at night when you're sleeping, your body says, "I can't build the necessary muscle, repair tissue, resynthesize glycogen, and do all those wonderful things on 800 calories. What do you expect of me? For goodness sake, eat some food if you're going to exercise like that!"

Stress also diminishes the usefulness of upper-end aerobic exercise. Research has shown that people who are stressed don't synthesize protein very well, meaning that they don't build or repair tissues as well. No matter how much protein they eat or how well balanced their diet, protein isn't used as well under stress. If you exercise at 80 percent of maximum, your body says, "I can't build good things in here because the stress is robbing my protein."

When is it smart to slow down?

The foregoing examples simply tell us that lots of people can benefit by exercising more gently. There are times when what seems like absurdly slow exercise is the best way to maintain and improve fitness. If you slow down, take it easy, think good thoughts (which helps to reduce stress), you'll repair better at night.

You don't have to be old, sick, or stressed to make good use of low-intensity (65–70 percent MHR) exercise. Everybody benefits from it. The smart exerciser uses low intensity as a basis, adding the high-intensity tricks of the last chapter when appropriate. The two are not contradictory; the wise reader will mix them and get the best of both.

How Often Should I Exercise?

When highly trained athletes increase their training from one session a day to two or more, there is often no improvement in their oxygen uptake. How can that be? The reason is that their first workout is so intense and so long that additional sessions just result in fatigue and overtraining.

The average person, in contrast, can add more workouts in a day quite easily. It makes me laugh to hear someone say, "Oh! you'll overtrain if you do two aerobic classes a day!" These people have obviously never met a fourteen-year-old boy who does aerobics, anaerobics, and all kinds of exercise fifteen or twenty times IN A SINGLE DAY. Aerobic exercise can be done frequently as long as you remember the rule — aerobic means not out of breath. Not-out-of-breath, true aerobic exercise can be done two, three, or four times a day. A high-level athlete exercising anaerobically can't be compared to the average person exercising gently. Aerobic class instructors might overtrain if they conduct two or three classes a day, but their students probably won't. The instructors have to put on a good show while calling out the moves. As a result, they are often exercising anaerobically while leading other people through a comfortable aerobic exercise.

Older people who have started exercising three or four times a week say, "I'm exercising more now than I ever did in my life." That probably isn't true. They don't remember how much they moved around when they were young. Kids don't sit on the beach; they play volleyball. They don't sit on the front lawn;

they roll and twist and play and throw things at each other. Kids are *always* moving. They don't say, "Gotta stop playing now, I might overtrain." People who are unfit or fat would be smart to imitate their little brothers and sisters. Short bouts of exercise are easier to face than thirty minutes of continuous jogging or cycling. A ten- or fifteen-minute walk around the block two or three times a day doesn't seem so bad.

> **The less intense the aerobic exercise, the more often you can do it — even five times a day.**

How often one should exercise, then, depends on the intensity of the exercise. The more intense the activity, the longer it takes the body to recover from it and the less often it should be performed.

Overtraining

When your level of fitness decreases even though you're exercising more, we say you are *overtraining*. Unfit or moderately trained people CAN overtrain, but it is more likely to happen to "jocks," simply because they spend more hours training and are less likely to give up. When a sedentary person or even an average athlete increases her exercise, she is more likely to suffer an injury before she gets the classic signs of overtraining. And if she does get those symptoms, she usually stops exercising. An athlete just keeps pushing herself.

A peculiar thing happens when we exercise too much. Many of the problems we were seeking to eliminate start cropping up again. If you exercise just enough, you tend to have fewer colds; exercise too much and you'll get more. Moderate exercise increases bone density; excessive exercise decreases it. Positive mood alterations are associated with daily exercise; mood disturbances erupt when you push yourself too hard.

Even though exercise is almost a magical remedy for ill health, if you overdo it, you'll produce risks rather than rewards. I have made the point repeatedly that the following three expressions are practically synonymous:

Health
Oxygen uptake
Fitness

Exercise done correctly improves all three. When overdone, exercise jeopardizes all three, as the graph on the next page

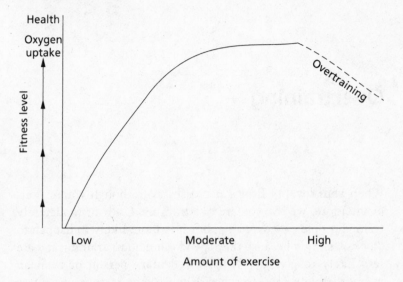

shows. The "overtraining syndrome" affects both your body and your mind. In general, you feel tired all the time, yet you sleep poorly. You seem to catch more colds. You don't look forward to your exercise sessions and, once in them, you aren't able to perform as well as you used to. Most of the time you're either angry or depressed. The list of problems is varied and, of course, you may not have all of them. But if you are experiencing four or five of the following symptoms, you could be in or approaching an overtrained state:

- Fatigue, lethargy
- Impaired performance
- Higher resting heart rate
- Slower reaction time
- Muscle pain, heavy-legged feeling
- Joint pain
- Sleep problems
- Loss of weight, drawn appearance
- Loss of appetite
- Poor coordination

- Irritability, depression, apathy
- Gastrointestinal disturbances, such as diarrhea
- Increased need for fluids during the night
- Elevated diastolic blood pressure

It amazes me that some people, thinking these symptoms are "good for me," continue to push themselves when their bodies are sending the clear message, "Hey! Enough already!" A friend of mine, whom I shall call Sue, is a case in point. She liked weightlifting so much she quit work for a while to train extra hard to be a competitive bodybuilder. She spent three to four hours every day lifting weights, and she ran for an hour in the evening. When I saw Sue about three months into her program, I was startled by her appearance. No doubt she was more muscular, but she looked awful. Her shapely buttocks had flattened, her rosy skin was sallow, and there were dark circles under her eyes. I asked her how she was doing.

> **Too much exercise can produce the same symptoms as too little exercise.**

"Frankly," she said, "I don't feel that well today. I'm really tired, I'm cranky, and I have diarrhea." Classic signs of overtraining. But Sue rationalized these signs away, claiming that the "toxins" in her body were being expelled, and if she continued her intense workouts, pretty soon she'd feel better. She eventually became too exhausted to continue. Her physician told her she must forgo *all* exercise for six months in order to recuperate. This is not a far-fetched or isolated example. People who ignore the symptoms of overtraining often require several months of recuperation. Even though Sue exercised more and more, her fitness decreased, her oxygen uptake decreased, AND her health decreased.

How to Avoid Overtraining

Too much exercise

Top athletes and their trainers minimize the possibility of over-training by manipulating the amount, intensity, and type of exercise. Typically they start the season with a lot of low-intensity work. As the season progresses, they exercise less often but more intensely. During this time the emphasis is on technique. Between seasons the players stay in shape with "active rest," engaging in low-key sports other than the sport they're training for.

You can apply these same principles to your daily routine. If you are a runner, go long distances at a slow pace on some days and short distances faster on others. If you feel you can't afford to take a day off from exercise, do an "active rest" activity such as hiking, bicycling, or swimming. Bodybuilders can achieve the same result by alternating long, gentle workouts with short, intense ones.

Most important, occasionally check your pace, as described in Covert's Home Fitness Test (page 175) and then apply the rule: if your pace is slowing down even though you're exercising more, then ease off — you're probably overtraining.

> **Alternate long, gentle exercise with short, hard workouts.**

Too little food

Loss of appetite is a typical sign of overtraining. Just when your muscles need calories and glycogen the most, you don't feel like eating. If you're exercising hard and long, be sure you get plenty of calories *and*, in particular, plenty of complex carbohydrates. Although the liver can make glycogen out of protein, it prefers to make it out of carbohydrate. While it's true that athletes need more protein if they're exercising intensely, they also need to be sure to eat plenty of fruits, vegetables, and other complex carbohydrates such as pastas and cereals. Otherwise the protein in the diet is used to replace glycogen instead of to repair muscle.

Not enough rest

Take your rest periods as seriously as you do your exercise. Muscle tissue doesn't grow stronger during exercise, it breaks down. It needs a period of rest to repair and build up. Back-to-back hard workouts mean constant muscle wear without tissue regeneration. When nine ultra-long-distance runners who participated in a seventeen-mile-a-day, ten-day race had their thighs measured before and after the race, the measurement actually *decreased*. You'd expect the quadriceps to get bigger after such an event, but they were smaller!

> **To avoid overtraining, never, ever run a marathon.**

Bodybuilders also find that a little rest pays off. A well-known female competitor once wrote an article describing the difficulty she was having trying to develop her biceps. She worked the muscle daily. Nothing happened. She increased the weight. No improvement. In frustration, she cut back on the weight and took every other day off. The poor muscle, finally getting a chance to repair, grew larger.

Finally, with tongue in cheek noted here, it's fine to train for a marathon, but you can avoid overtraining if you never actually run in one. Researchers have found that among people who train for a marathon but decide not to run it, only 2 percent become sick, compared with 13 percent of those who run the twenty-six-mile event. Associating illness with marathons is sort of ridiculous, but there is a clear-cut relationship between overtraining and sickness. People who run more than sixty miles per week are twice as likely to become ill as those who run only twenty miles per week.

Effects of Excessive versus Moderate Exercise

System	Moderate Exercise	Excessive Exercise
Heart/circulatory	Control of blood pressure in people with mild hypertension	Increase in diastolic blood pressure
	Decrease in resting heart rate	Rise in resting heart rate
	Lowered risk of heart disease	Increased risk of cardiac arrest in high-risk people
Musculoskeletal	Increased muscle strength	Injuries from fatigued muscles
		Muscle atrophy
	Prevention of bone loss	Loss of bone mineral in nonmenstruating female athletes
		Increased risk of osteoarthritis

System	Moderate Exercise	Excessive Exercise
Immune	Improvement of immune system function	Depressed immune function
	Fewer colds and flus	Increased risk of colds, flu
		Poor healing of scratches
Sleep	Tendency to feel more awake with fewer hours of sleep	Sleep disturbances: harder to fall asleep, wake often during night, hard to wake up in morning
Psychological	Elevated mood	Generalized apathy
	Decreased anxiety and depression	Lethargy
	Improved short-term mental cognition	Depression
		Anger
		Exercise addiction

How to Get Fit Fast

If you look at the following list of exercises and the number of minutes I suggest for each, you can see that you have to walk a long time to get the same benefits as you'd get from a short session of cross-country skiing. Why is that? Some people think the difference comes from the amount of effort required. Not so! Even if walking is done with lots of effort and cross-country skiing done with little effort, the difference is still seen. It's the *amount of muscle* involved in the exercise that matters.

How Long Should You Exercise?

Exercise	Minimum time required for systemic response
Walking	40 minutes
Bicycling, indoor	25 minutes
Bicycling, outdoor	20 minutes
Swimming	20 minutes
Jogging	15 minutes
Rowing	15 minutes
Cross-country skiing	12 minutes

When we walk on the level, our legs are almost straight, so little muscle is required to swing them. Walking is a good exercise, but you have to do it for a long time before your body feels the need to adapt to it. Biking, on the other hand, involves more muscle even though you're sitting. It requires the quadriceps, hamstrings, and sometimes the abdominal muscles as you pull on the handlebar. Because it uses more muscle, more deeply, biking brings about a systemic response more quickly. After twenty or twenty-five minutes your body knows you've been exercising and responds with chemical changes in the heart, blood, bone, and a host of other areas.

> **When you exercise, the more muscle you use, the less long you gotta do it!**

Jogging uses even more muscle. I laugh when I hear claims that walking and jogging are the same exercise. That's ridiculous! You need much more muscle to jog — for the added speed, for vertical movement (up-and-down bouncing), for deeper breathing, even for unconscious balance adjustment. There's no comparison between the effort needed to jog fifteen minutes and the effort to walk fifteen minutes. Don't let anyone tell you they are the same. Jogging uses so much muscle you don't have to do it long to get a whole-body response from it.

Of course, you can *make* walking a harder exercise than jogging, can't you? Put a fifty-pound pack on your back, then hike up Pike's Peak. Now you're using much more muscle. When people have joint problems from jogging, they can switch to backpack walking, hill walking, even to using ski pole–type walking sticks so you're using enough extra musculature to get the same systemic improvement as in jogging but with reduced trauma.

Cross-country skiing uses practically every muscle you have — arms, legs, back, thighs, buttocks, everything. In just twelve minutes your body says, "Wow! he's really exercising! I'd better make my muscles and organs healthier as fast as I can!"

Swimming appears to be a multimuscle activity, but in fact it is mostly an upper-body exercise. It uses the arms with their small muscles much more than the legs with their big muscles. In doing the crawl, you swing your legs much as you do when walking. There is little of the pumping you must do in running or cross-country skiing. Swimming is an excellent exercise, but you need to swim for at least twenty minutes to get systemic changes.

I've only touched on the common exercises. You may be wondering about roller blading, or trampolining, or stair climbing, or step aerobics, or something else. I could devote pages to each exercise, but it all boils down to — how much muscle are you using? You can use a lot or a little muscle with something like a stair climber. I've seen people on stair machines who look like they've invented a new tiptoe dance and others who really go at it. And the minutes listed for each form of exercise are only guidelines. If you've got a way of walking that uses a lot of muscle — race walking, for instance — then you don't need to spend as much time doing it. Just remember my rule — "The more muscle you use, the less long you gotta do it!"

Bicycling versus Cross-Country Skiing

Let's compare a stationary bicycle to a cross-country ski machine. Bicycling uses mostly the quadriceps. I'm sure we've all felt that lactic acid burn when bicycling uphill. The same thing happens on a stationary bike. It's very easy to get lactate in the thigh muscles by pedaling a little too fast or tightening the tension. Bicycling uses a limited amount of muscle and tends to use it at a very high level of intensity. In contrast, cross-country skiing uses all the muscles at a much lower intensity. Both exercises are good — but there is a very important point to be made here. As I have shown in previous chapters, if you use a muscle at a high level of intensity, the exercise tends to become anaerobic, making lactic acid. What does lactic acid in the muscle indicate? That the muscle is burning sugar, which is what can happen when you use a bicycle. If you push yourself to the point that you start to get the lactic acid burn, you're burning only sugar and not fat.

It's harder to push yourself on a cross-country ski machine to the point of producing lactic acid because instead of pushing one muscle much harder, you push many muscles just a little harder. Now the limiting factor is your breathing and your heart rate rather than lactic acid in the muscle. As a result, you're much more likely to be burning fat in those muscles instead of sugar.

Let's say you use a cross-country ski machine one day and a

stationary bicycle the next day, each time exercising at exactly the same heart rate. For many years researchers thought that if you exercised at the same pulse or heart rate, you were doing the same amount of work, burning the same number of calories, and losing fat at the same rate. Now you can see that is not true. The bicycle exercise, using a little muscle at high intensity, burns sugar. The skiing exercise, using a lot of muscle at low intensity, burns fat. The difference in total calories burned might be no more than 5 percent, not worth talking about. However, the cross-country ski machine may raise the percentage of fat burned by 30 percent.

**Do some aerobic exercises
burn more fat than others?**

To analyze any aerobic exercise, ask yourself, "How much muscle am I using?" If you're using lots of muscle at a low level, you're more likely to burn off body fat.

Cross Training

If your left arm is in a cast for two months, the muscles will shrivel, or atrophy, a bit. Whether the arm is broken or completely healthy, total inactivity for two months is going to make it weaker. Now suppose you lift weights with the other arm for those two months. What happens? The casted arm will atrophy less. This phenomenon was what the term "cross training" originally described. It's hard to believe that exercising one arm affects muscle in the other, but it does. Atrophy can be diminished by exercising the opposite limb.

What if you aren't wearing a cast and both arms are healthy, but you lift weights with the left arm only? The right arm will get stronger — not as strong as the left arm, but it does get stronger. Contralateral exercise not only prevents the wasting of muscle in an opposite injured limb, it also stimulates muscle growth and strength in an opposite uninjured, but unused, limb. The nerves that carry sensations up one limb to the spine connect with nerves that carry sensations down into the opposing limb. The sensations and stimuli occurring in the exercised limb are transcribed by wire to the other limb.

Let's go further. Will changes occur in the left arm if the right leg is exercised? That's a really far-out idea. It's harder to prove in laboratory studies, but there is an effect. It's easier to understand when you realize that exercising the right leg also affects the liver, heart, and blood. In other words, the exercise has systemic effects; the changes in arm muscle are only part of a bigger picture. When we exercise the right leg, the changes to the left arm are not neurological as they are in opposite limbs but, rather, systemic. Apparently exercising a lower limb hard can bring about changes in the blood, liver, and lungs that allow the upper limbs to perform better. The improvements are not limited to systemic changes; there are local changes as well. For example, enzymes increase in nontrained muscles. If a person started using a stationary bicycle, being careful to keep her upper body as still as possible, after six months we would find increases in oxygen-dependent enzymes in the muscles of her upper body.

> **Exercising the left leg makes the right leg stronger — even if the right leg is in a cast.**

Turn the experiment upside down; do legs respond to arm exercise? If the right arm exercises while the left leg is in a cast, there is little or no cross-training effect because the arm muscles are too small to demand much of the heart, lungs, or blood. Systemic changes are minimal. The huge leg muscles, in contrast, produce significant systemic effects.

Cross training from one arm or leg to the opposite arm or leg occurs because of nerve connections; from one leg to an arm it occurs because of systemic changes. But you do not get cross training from an arm to a leg because there are no nerve connections and the arm muscle is too small to produce systemic effects.

Nowadays, the term "cross training" is used in a much broader sense, stretching its narrow scientific meaning. Runners "cross train" by cycling, and swimmers "cross train" by lifting weights. Are they really cross training? You bet they are. The more trained muscle a person has, the greater the crossover response in unused muscle.

This also means that if you're fat and want to increase your butter-burning machinery, the more muscles you train, the more working *and* nonworking muscles will be involved in fat burning.

Cross training offers an additional bonus during competition. The more muscles you train, the more oxygen-dependent enzymes there will be to process lactic acid. Muscles that are heavily used in that sport produce lactic acid, which can then be processed by aerobically developed muscles that are not being overused during the sport. Laboratory studies show that runners who add aerobic arm training to their program have a slower — and smaller — rise in lactate levels during racing. Moreover, there is a faster return to normal levels after the race is over.

> **Older people would be smart to use the cross-training tricks of athletes.**

Athletes have been using the contralateral limb effect for years. The shame is that nonathletes make so little use of it, and the biggest shame is that older people don't know that it works for them. As you get into your sixties and beyond, it's harder to retain muscle mass. Old folks lose muscle not only because they exercise less but also because it takes them longer to repair and rebuild muscle after exercise. Older people should use the cross-training trick routinely to maintain muscle mass and strength.

Natural Exercise versus Machines

You'd think that a stationary bicycle would be just as effective for getting fit as an outdoor bicycle, but it isn't. People using road bikes get fitter than people using stationary bikes. For one thing, outdoor bicycling is more fun, so you're likely to keep at it longer. Not many of us continue to pedal a stationary bike after the timer bell goes off. We leap off the bike with a sigh of relief and head for the shower. Outdoor cyclists may find it harder to get started, but once they do, they go on longer because they're having a good time. It's a sport as well as an exercise. However, it's not just a matter of how long we do it. There's another subtle thing that makes natural exercise more effective than machine simulators.

Weightlifters were the first to learn that using free weights — barbells and dumbbells — trained muscles quicker and better than machines. When this idea was first rumored, you can imagine how the equipment manufacturers responded. Hearing professional weightlifters state that they preferred free weights to machines, the manufacturers were quick to present research trying to prove that machines were better. In the end the weightlifters were right. Why? Because balance is a more important factor in exercise than had been realized. When we balance a weight we use more of a given muscle; different fibers and levels of the muscle are brought into play to lift and balance at the same time.

Balancing not only adds to the fun on an outdoor bike, cross-country skis, or roller skates, it adds a cross-training effect.

Sitting on a stationary bike requires no balance. The left leg simply pushes, with minimal cross signals to the right leg. But if the left leg is pushing while the right leg is balancing, as when you're biking outdoors, you're actually training and exercising both legs while pushing with one.

> **There's nothing like that warm glow after a day of cross-country skiing — on a machine in your basement!**

Even running outdoors requires more balance than running on a treadmill, especially if you run on a trail instead of an asphalt surface. You have to zig and zag, jump over little sticks in the road, and sometimes run uphill, which also gives the wind-sprint effect. It's very difficult to get any of that balancing effect on a treadmill, and obviously it's difficult to do a wind sprint on a treadmill unless you speed it up occasionally.

I'm not saying that machines are no good. They are particularly good for beginners because they lessen the chances of injury. They make it easier for a beginner to get started. They're great for bad weather and for times when it's impossible to get out. It's just that outdoor exercise becomes more than exercise. It becomes a fun sport so you do more of it, and that, along with the balancing effect, makes you fitter faster.

5

Training

This is the section that fat people might skip, thinking that it's not for them. Don't skip it!! Most of the best stuff we know about getting rid of fat comes from research on athletes and their training.

The Three Sources of Energy

Fat People and Slow Metabolism

Wind-Sprint Theory

How to Do Wind Sprints

Wind Sprints — for Very Fat People?

Training at Altitude

Is Performance Improved by Breathing Pure Oxygen?

Athlete's Blood

The Three Sources of Energy

I have explained that muscles contract only if there are ATP-matches inside the muscle cell. I showed how phosphorus breaks off from the matches, providing energy to the cell, and pointed out that for the cell to contract repeatedly, the ATP-matches must have some fresh phosphorus put back on so that they can be used over and over. The more intense the exercise, the faster the ATP-matches are used and the harder it is to remake new ones to keep up with the demand. Intense exercise like sprinting exhausts the supply of ATP-matches in ten seconds or less, forcing the runner to gasp to a halt. In contrast, gentle long-distance exercise uses the ATP-matches slowly, so the muscle cell has time to get energy from fats and sugars and to refurbish the matches as fast as they are used.

Muscle has three separate biochemical tricks — energy sources — for rebuilding ATP, depending on the intensity of exercise:

One for ten-second sprints and energy bursts
One for long, slow distance
One for effort intermediate between the other two, middle-distance exercise

If you can learn the basic principles of each of the three energy sources, you can design exercise specifically to meet your goals. You can train for sprints, basketball, marathon running, or simply — fat loss.

The Aerobic System

When you run aerobically, as long as there is plenty of oxygen, ATP will be manufactured from the breakdown of fat and sugar. This system can produce almost limitless amounts of ATP. If you need energy for endurance exercise, count on the aerobic system.

The Lactate System

In contrast, when you run anaerobically, the lack of oxygen not only turns off fat burning, it also blocks pyruvate from entering the Krebs cycle. Pyruvate builds up and is converted to lactic acid, or lactate. The only ATP produced comes from the burning of sugar halfway; thus the amount of energy produced is limited. But the beauty of this system is that it doesn't have to wait for oxygen, so the ATP is produced very fast. If you need fresh ATP in a hurry, the lactate system will kick in to burn lots of sugar molecules quickly. You will get quick energy — but it won't last.

The Creatine-Phosphate System

There is a third (and last) method to build fresh ATP. Each muscle cell contains another chemical with hot phosphorus on the end. It, too, can be likened to a kitchen match. The wooden part of the match is creatine; when its phosphorus is in place, it's called creatine-phosphate or creatine-P. If you want to do a super-hard, fast sprint, creatine-P is waiting right in the cell. It doesn't need enzymes to produce energy; it explodes as needed, releasing energy fast enough to rebuild ATP no matter how fast you run. As the phosphorus explodes on a creatine-match, the

**The Aerobic System
(endurance exercise)**

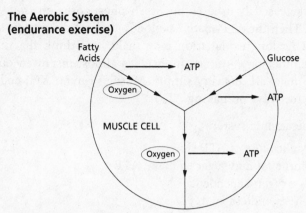

**The Lactate System
(stop-and-go exercise)**

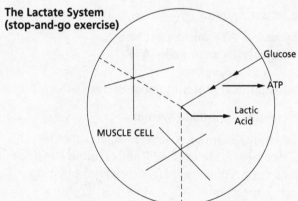

**The Creatine-Phosphate
System
(intense exercise)**

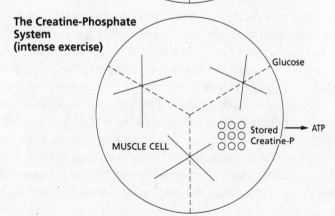

energy released is used to put fresh phosphorus on the ATP-match. Then the ATP-match explodes, making the muscle contract. This long explanation may make you think that it's a slow, cumbersome system. In fact, it's almost instantaneous.

Let's make all this very simple. Muscles run on ATP, and we have three ways of making ATP.

1. The aerobic system

   - Makes lots of ATP slowly
   - Burns fat and sugar to make ATP
   - Is oxygen-dependent
   - Gives endless energy

2. The lactate system

   - Makes less ATP but does it fast
   - Burns only sugar to make ATP
   - Requires no oxygen
   - Yields up to seven minutes of energy

3. The creatine-phosphate system

   - Makes small amounts of ATP super, super fast
   - ATP comes from stored ATP and creatine-P inside muscle
   - Does not need oxygen, fat, or sugar to function
   - Lasts ten seconds

We can now divide our sports activities into three levels and train specifically for any one. Creatine-P is for intense sprints, ten seconds or less, such as a hundred-yard dash. At this intensity, the ATP present in cells is gobbled up in three seconds, and in the next seven seconds, creatine-P creates more ATP. Both sources are gone in ten seconds. The limiting factor, then, is the quantity of creatine-P in the cell. At the end of a one-hundred-yard dash, it isn't lack of oxygen or lack of glucose or the pain of lactic acid that stops you — it's lack of creatine-P. For such a sport, packing extra creatine-P in your muscles is essential.

For events longer than the one-hundred-yard dash and shorter than a mile, lasting ten seconds to seven minutes, it is the lactate system that produces energy. Pre-existing ATP is used up in three seconds, then the creatine-P is exhausted, and the rest of the event is dependent on the lactate system. The limiting factor this time is either lactic acid pain or running out of glucose. Training for sports in this range involves getting more glucose into the muscle and teaching the muscle to get rid of the lactate. Oxygen isn't used for either the lactate system or the creatine-P system, so the breathlessness you experience is not really what makes you stop.

> **Force yourself to learn the three energy systems — even if you're only interested in losing weight.**

For sports exercises lasting longer than seven minutes, oxygen is the critical factor; hence the word "aerobic." Such exercise may last for many hours, with the slow oxidation of fat and sugar supplying almost all of the ATP-matches. Training the aerobic system focuses on three tasks: getting more oxygen into the cell, building the cellular enzymes that "spark" oxygen to combine with fat and sugar, and not running out of glycogen kindling. Even though fat is the primary fuel of the aerobic system, fat is never the limiting factor; it's the glycogen supply that limits endurance events. Marathoners hit the wall when they run out of glycogen. Nobody ever runs out of fat! A mere pound of fat translates into 3,500 calories of energy. Even a skinny runner has more than enough fat to fuel a twenty-six-mile marathon.

Understanding the three systems discussed in this chapter will allow you to design an effective training regimen. You can train for sprints, middle-distance events, or marathons. It will help you understand when and what to eat. It gives you a basis for choosing the right length and intensity of your workouts. Even if your only interest is losing body fat effectively, understanding these three systems is mandatory.

Please! Read the chapter again, take a piece of paper, and see if you can draw and explain the three systems to a friend without cheating. If your friend doesn't understand your explanation, you probably don't understand it either. Excuse me for acting like a college professor, but this is the kind of material that will guide you for a lifetime.

Fat People and Slow Metabolism

With all this talk about energy systems, a fat person might conclude that this book is just for jocks. If he did, he'd be missing an important point.

There are people who don't eat excessively yet get fat easily and have a terrible time losing their fat. They assume that something is wrong with their metabolism. Thinking that they are overeating, they go on a diet, but eventually they realize that they stay fat even though they are eating less than some of their friends.

If you're one of these people, read the previous chapter on the three sources of energy. The problem with your metabolism ought to hit you between the eyes. If you aren't getting rid of fat, your aerobic energy system isn't working. When fat molecules arrive in your muscles, they're not burned properly. You don't need a diet, you need to raise your fat metabolism. What conditions are needed to make muscles burn fat? The muscle needs fat-burning enzymes, and it needs oxygen for those enzymes to function. Together, the oxygen and enzymes burn fatty acids, producing ATP. Exercise builds up those enzymes and increases the muscle's ability to take up oxygen. To "speed up" your metabolism, you need to speed up your aerobic energy system. Only exercise, *not* diet, can do that.

The aerobic system also "speeds up" metabolism *after* exercise. Have you ever wondered why you continue to breathe deeply after you stop exercising? Why doesn't your breathing go back to normal immediately? If your muscle cells no longer need lots of oxygen, why do you keep breathing in lots of oxygen? The answer is that the ATP-matches need to be replaced pronto, and that requires oxygen. In the first few minutes after exercise, when you are still breathing quite deeply, the oxygen is combined with sugar and fat to make the necessary energy to put the phosphorus back on the ATP-matches.

> **You produce energy in three ways, but only one of those ways burns fat.**

For the next hour or so, you continue to breathe faster than normal. The muscles are now using the oxygen to replenish their glycogen supplies. Obviously, the type, intensity, and duration of exercise influences the amount of glycogen to be restored. The aerobic system is the only energy system operating during recovery from exercise. The more jobs it has to do after exercise, the more metabolism is elevated. That's why the post-exercise period helps you lose fat.

Metabolism isn't as complicated as some people want you to think. Do you burn fat in your muscle or not? If you don't, read the last chapter to find out what it takes to get your muscles to do so. You need to ask yourself, "Why doesn't my aerobic energy system work? My body produces energy three ways, and only one of those three ways uses fat." If you are fat, that is what you need to work on, not another diet.

Wind-Sprint Theory

Each of the three energy systems works only as long as its energy source lasts. Thus the creatine-phosphate system lasts seconds, the lactate system lasts minutes, and the aerobic system can sometimes last for hours. But if you do *intermittent* exercise, the different systems can be manipulated so that the benefits of one system override the drawbacks of another.

Suppose you run as fast as you can for one minute. After the first ten seconds of the run, the ATP and creatine-P in the muscles are all used up; the lactate system gets you through the last fifty seconds. As a result, your legs are screaming in pain from lactic acid buildup. You are exhausted at the end and need several minutes to recover.

Now suppose you do the same run again, but this time you run as fast as you can for ten seconds, then rest for thirty seconds, run again for ten, rest again for thirty, and so on until your total running time, as before, is one minute. The run is just as long and just as intense, but now you're not nearly as tired as you were after the continuous one-minute run.

When you do the run in spurts of ten seconds, creatine-P is the predominant energy system used. This system depletes very rapidly, but it is also replenished rapidly if you slow down enough for the aerobic system to refuel it. In a series of short sprints, supplies of ATP and creatine-P are drained during the ten seconds of running, then restored during the thirty seconds of rest. As a result, the lactate system is used very little, there

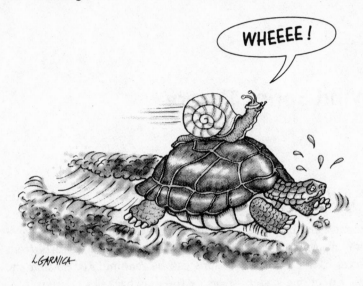

WHEEEE !

L GARNICA

Turtle Wind Sprints

is no lactic acid buildup, and therefore you feel considerably less fatigued.

This is only one application of wind-sprint theory, but it illustrates the advantage of slow/fast exercising. So that we can discuss it further without confusion, let's call the fast, intense part the sprint and the slower, less intense part the recovery.

These two parts can be manipulated in several ways:

1. Intensity of sprint
2. Duration of sprint
3. Intensity of recovery
4. Duration of recovery

In the old days everyone did wind sprints, or interval training, pretty much the same way. They ran as hard as they could for as long as they could, walked until they got their breath back, then did another sprint, another walk, and so on to exhaustion.

Today we've found that by manipulating the four variables listed, you can specifically train each energy system. A sprinter can train the creatine-phosphate system so that it lasts a little longer than ten seconds. A middle-distance athlete can do a different kind of wind sprint to develop a higher tolerance to lactic acid. Endurance athletes can manipulate the sprint and recovery in yet another way to develop the aerobic system to greatest advantage.

> **Sprinters, marathoners, even fat people can benefit from wind sprints — if they learn how to do them right.**

A fat person, reading all this training talk, might decide to skip this chapter, but please pay attention to what I just said. *By doing wind sprints a certain way, the aerobic system — the fat-burning system — can be trained to work better.*

Let's go to the next chapter, on the specifics of interval training, and see how each of the four variables can be manipulated.

How to Do Wind Sprints

There are many ways to interval train. You can sprint very fast and then walk. You can sprint very fast and then slow down to a jog. You can sprint for just a few seconds or, by slowing down a bit, go for three or four minutes. Similarly, the rest periods between sprints can be brief or extended. By changing the four components of interval training (intensity of sprint, duration of sprint, intensity of rest, duration of rest) an athlete can train the specific energy system he needs to develop for his sport.

To become a better sprinter, for instance, you need to train the creatine-P system by doing hard short sprints followed by long walks. The sprinter needs to be completely aerobic, breathing comfortably, before his next sprint so that ATP and creatine-P are fully restored. The muscles say, "If he's going to sprint that hard, we have to make more ATP than normal between the sprints." They can do that only if the rest period is completely aerobic. We call this a "rest" recovery.

A basketball player, tennis player, soccer player, or middle-distance runner wants to train his lactate system. Think about the way these athletes play. Sometimes they sprint all out, and sometimes they trot comfortably. They need to train in such a way that the lactic acid buildup is delayed. To do this, they need to slow down only to a jog, a "work" recovery that doesn't quite get their breath back, then sprint again *before* they have completely recovered. Their ATP and creatine-P are only partially replenished, so the next sprint uses more of the lactate system for energy. The muscles learn to handle greater and greater loads of lactic acid with less fatigue.

Finally, the endurance athlete can also benefit from interval training in developing his aerobic system. Since wind sprints are inherently anaerobic, you may be wondering, "How can you train the aerobic system by doing anaerobic work?" The answer is that aerobic enzymes increase in response to the tasks required of them *during recovery*. During recovery, aerobic enzymes not only replace ATP and creatine-P, they also process lactic acid. The enzymes say, "If he's going to sprint every now and then, we need to grow so that we can make new ATP faster and get rid of lactic acid faster." In other words, the aerobic enzymes increase in response to anaerobic stress. *But* — they only function under aerobic conditions. Therefore, to develop the aerobic system, the athlete must exercise aerobically during the recovery period. The neat thing about training the aerobic system with wind sprints is that one of the other two systems gets trained as well. If you slow down to a jog during recovery, the lactate and aerobic systems are trained. If you slow down to a walk so that your breath comes back more quickly, the creatine-P and aerobic systems develop. In either case, don't do the next sprint until you are *completely* recovered from the last.

If you feel muddled at this point, just remember these two rules:

1. If you are training to be a sprinter or a long-distance runner, you need to completely get your breath back during the rest periods.
2. If you are training for middle-distance and stop-and-go sports, you should *not* get your breath back completely during the rest periods.

There are differences in the sprint part as well. For the sprinter the sprints are very short, very intense, and very frequent. They become a little longer, less frequent, and less intense for the middle-distance athlete, and still longer, fewer, and milder for the endurance athlete.

Types of Interval Training

System trained	Intensity of sprint	Duration of sprint	Intensity of recovery	Duration of recovery	Sets/ Repetitions
Creatine-phosphate (sprinting)	High (95–100% MHR)	10–20 sec.	Rest recovery	3 times as long as sprint	5 sets/10 reps each set
Lactate (middle distance; stop-and-go)	Moderately high (85–90% MHR)	1–2 min.	Work recovery	2 times as long as sprint	2–4 sets/4 reps each set
Aerobic (long distance)	Moderate (80–85% MHR)	3–5 min.	Rest recovery	½ as long as sprint	1 set/3 reps

From the table you can see that the sprint is not necessarily all-out in intensity but should be somewhere between 85 percent and 95 percent of maximum. A sprinter would push himself to nearly maximum (95 percent), but an endurance runner would run only slightly faster than his usual pace (85 percent instead of 80 percent).

Coaches are extremely precise in determining exactly how fast they want their competition athletes to run during the sprint. These athletes need to work hard enough to tax whichever specific system they want to train without becoming too fatigued. If you are not into competition but just want to get fitter, don't worry too much about intensity. Just run faster than usual but not so fast that you can't complete the recommended number of sets and repetitions.

In the last chapter I said that fat people can also profit from wind sprints. Typically we urge out-of-shape people to not get out of breath when they exercise, but wind sprints are a special case. Wind sprints are THE fastest way to improve fitness and increase fat-burning enzymes. A fat person has so few of these enzymes that hours of walking may not stimulate their growth. Occasionally they need to be "shocked" into increasing their numbers. A fat person should follow the guidelines in the table for training the aerobic system. For him the "sprint" might be only a fast walk, something that gets him slightly out of breath. If he does this two or three times during a thirty-minute walk and does it every third or fourth exercise session, the muscles say, "Hey! we're fine when he walks, but every now and then he speeds up. We need to make more fat-burning enzymes so he can still burn fat when he speeds up. When he slows down we can use the extra fat-burning enzymes to replace the ATP-matches faster."

The frequency of interval training depends on the sport. A nonendurance athlete, such as a sprinter or weightlifter, usually trains only three times a week, and nearly all of his workouts are high-intensity, interval-type training. An endurance athlete, a recreational athlete, or a fat or out-of-shape person should be exercising four to five days a week at low intensities. For this type of program, interval training should be used only once or, at most, twice a week. Those who play the in-between, lactic-acid-producing sports should do interval training on one or two days and aerobic workouts the rest of the time.

Wind Sprints — for Very Fat People?

It's hard to picture two very overweight people discussing wind sprints. Overweight people usually talk about diet or some other kind of self-denial. It's tough enough to be a hundred pounds overweight without thinking about doing wind sprints, which are typically associated with athletes. However, I've emphasized several times that the intensity of wind sprints improves fitness quickly. And it's high fitness that allows you to burn lots of fat.

If you are fat, you are probably thinking, "I don't care how much theory you spout favoring wind sprints. With all my surplus fat, I am not going outdoors and sprint. I would look ridiculous and probably kill myself."

Well, calm down; let me explain something. Using the word "sprint" can be confusing. In the "wind sprint" context it doesn't mean run as fast as you can; it means go a little faster than comfortable. And you are probably doing that occasionally already.

In other words, fat people often do wind sprints without realizing it. Walking up a small hill is likely to make a one-hundred-pound-overweight person out of breath, but no one would say, "Look at that person doing a wind sprint." Yet he *is* doing a kind of wind sprint. Remember, the principle is to go fast enough to get a little out of breath and then return to the pre-sprint pace. Overweight people can apply this by adding a short jog, or a short uphill stretch in the middle of an otherwise comfortable aerobic walk. They will become fitter much more quickly than the person who simply walks longer distances or walks more often. It's better to do a walk with occasional short bursts of effort in the middle than to walk longer or more frequently.

> **If you want to lose fat, you need to add little spurts of intensity to your walk.**

It's too bad that the thought of wind sprints is a turn-off to fat people, because they can derive as much benefit from them as athletes. Even though the exercise research and information come from studies on athletes, the principles apply equally well to people who are overweight.

Training at Altitude

People who live at high altitudes find it much easier to exercise when they come down from their mountain, largely because they have more red blood cells. Since red blood cells carry oxygen to the tissues, you could say mountain people have turbocharged blood. Knowing this, some athletes go on weekend excursions to the mountains, hoping that the altitude will pep up their red blood cell levels so they can run faster in an upcoming race. Unfortunately, it takes more than a few days for red blood cells to increase to the levels found in people who live in the mountains. It's a long process.

Here's what happens. The air at higher altitudes has less oxygen. When oxygen in the blood is low, it triggers the secretion of a hormone that stimulates the bone marrow to produce more red blood cells. This hormone is formed within a few hours of breathing thin air, but the new red blood cells don't appear in circulation for five days. Athletes who train at altitude for two or three days can't hope to increase their red blood cell count in so short a time. It takes two to three weeks before there are enough new red blood cells to make any difference and several months before the increase is complete.

Suppose you decide to spend a couple of months training at high altitude to raise your red blood cell count. Will your performance improve? Possibly, but not if you're super fit to start with. When the Olympic Games were held in Mexico City (7,800 feet) a few years ago, many elite athletes prepared by training at high altitude. Unfortunately, their performance didn't

improve as much as they hoped: their high level of fitness actually worked against them. The thin air at high altitude prevented them from exerting maximum effort, so they couldn't
exercise with their usual intensity or duration. They simply
couldn't train as hard in the mountains as they could at sea
level.

If an average runner, on the other hand, trained at high altitude for a few months, she would be able to run faster and
longer at lower altitudes. But the effect is temporary. Once she
descended to sea level, all those extra red blood cells would be
lost in as little as three days.

> **"Will training at altitude help me
> perform better when I return to
> sea level?"**

There are poignant stories of Bolivian peasants who live all
their lives at 14,000 feet. Their bodies become so adapted to the
low level of oxygen that the older residents find it impossible
to leave. If an older villager leaves his home to visit relatives at
sea level, his body adjusts to the lower altitude by losing some
of the adaptations necessary to survive at high altitude. When
he returns home, his body doesn't respond quickly enough to
the altitude and he dies.

The point is, even people who spend their lives in high-altitude environments lose the adaptation very quickly at sea level.
High-altitude training may help if you run the race within hours
after leaving the mountains, but it doesn't work that well for
most situations.

You would think that because fit people use oxygen more
efficiently than unfit people they would have no trouble adjust-
ing to high altitude during a weekend skiing or backpacking trip
in the mountains. Not so! Fit people perform better both at sea
level and at altitude, but their performance decreases in the

same proportion as it does for unfit people who exercise in thin air. Fitness doesn't seem to confer any special protection from the dizziness and nausea that we often experience at altitude.

If you're planning a weekend trip to the mountains, don't plan any strenuous activity for the first few hours after you arrive. Drive up the night before if you can, putting off hiking or skiing until the next morning. Don't try to run at the same speed you're used to at sea level. Find a pace that has you breathing at the same depth and rate as during your usual exercise. Your usual eight-minute-a-mile pace may take ten minutes at high altitude.

Endurance aerobic activities are more affected by altitude than are sprinting or anaerobic sports. This makes sense — endurance and aerobic activities require more oxygen. The major problem is oxygen insufficiency, and since anaerobic sports don't use as much oxygen, you don't notice fatigue as quickly as you do with aerobic sports. Downhill skiers, who use energy in short bursts, don't notice the altitude effects as much as cross-country skiers.

Is Performance Improved by Breathing Pure Oxygen?

Tests on athletes breathing oxygen-enriched air show that they have greater endurance, a lower heart rate, and a smaller accumulation of lactic acid throughout an exercise.

We all know that the power and performance of a small car engine can be tremendously improved by extra oxygen. That's what turbochargers do; they ram extra air through the carburetor into the engine. Similarly, when we huff and puff we are trying to cram in more oxygen. By breathing supplemental oxygen, we send more oxygen to working muscles, enabling them to work harder with less effort. Mountaineers climb better if they use oxygen tanks. Even untrained hikers can climb better if they have supplemental oxygen. In fact, we can go even further. If a very fat, sick person barely able to walk were taken to a high altitude, he also would perform better with supplemental oxygen.

While it is pretty clear that breathing supplemental oxygen during an event improves performance, it doesn't seem to help when used before an event or during intermissions. We've all seen football players with oxygen masks clamped to their faces while they rest on the sidelines. Does that superoxygenate their blood so they can run faster or push harder? No! Athletes who claim that supplemental oxygen improves their game are experiencing a placebo effect.

Athlete's Blood

If you whirl a tube of blood in a centrifuge, it settles into two distinct layers. At the bottom is a thick, sludgy layer that is mostly red blood cells. Floating on top is a yellowish, clear liquid called plasma. Plasma is mainly water with a few salts, fats, proteins, and carbohydrates dissolved in it. Normally we have in our bodies about five liters of blood (approximately five quarts for those of you who don't think metric). Of that, the plasma volume is around three liters, or quarts, and the red blood cell volume is about two liters. The ratio of the cellular part of blood to the liquid plasma part is called the hematocrit. Normal hematocrit is 45 percent; that is, 45 percent of blood is made up of red and white blood cells and 55 percent is plasma.

People who exercise regularly have more plasma; increases of 12 to 20 percent in volume are routine. Exercise flushes out proteins into the plasma, and this has an osmotic (water-attracting) effect. Water is pulled into the blood from tissues and intracellular spaces, making it more watery. In this thinned state, the blood flows more rapidly and more easily through vessels so that blood pressure is reduced. Exercised blood is like wine; sedentary blood is more like spaghetti sauce. That's an exaggeration, but it helps you visualize the difference.

As a result of this exercise-induced dilution, the heart is able to pump more blood with less pressure. Technically, we say that the increase in plasma volume allows for an increase in stroke volume; that is, the heart's output per stroke is increased.

An increase in plasma volume also helps regulate body heat.

More fluid means that the blood can carry more heat from the body's core to the skin surface, where it can escape into the air.

In addition to a higher volume of plasma, people who exercise a lot have more red blood cells. Whenever tissues need more oxygen, the bone marrow turns up its production of red blood cells. Living at high altitude stimulates the synthesis of red blood cells. Exercise also gears up production. Athletes have up to 7 million red blood cells per cubic millimeter of blood, compared to 5 million in the average person.

> **Regular exercise makes your blood more watery.**

We have, then, in the athlete an increase in both plasma volume and red blood cells. Yet when his blood is tested, he's often told he has a low hematocrit because the increase in plasma volume is greater than the increase in red blood cells. Even though the red blood cell count is higher than normal, it is disproportionately low compared to plasma volume. Red blood cells transport iron, and when a doctor sees a low hematocrit, he thinks, "Oh-oh, this guy might be anemic." But if the guy happens to be an athlete, the doctor says, "I need to do more tests than just the hematocrit." He knows that in about 50 percent of athletes with low hematocrit there's nothing wrong. They have pseudoanemia or "dilutional anemia."

Even though pseudoanemia is common in people who exercise a lot, real anemia does occur, particularly in highly trained athletes. Despite having normal or greater amounts of red blood cells, they may be low in iron, a condition that is somehow associated with very strenuous activity. Since iron depletion is more prevalent in runners than in cyclists, rowers, or swimmers, it may be that impact stress causes the breakdown of red blood cells. Iron might also be lost because of copious sweating, increased stress hormones, or muscle damage and subsequent leakage of iron-containing myoglobin. Also, many long-distance runners avoid eating meats, relying more on whole grains. Grains not only have less iron, it is also less available to the body than the iron in meat. Whatever the reason, many long-distance runners take iron supplements as a precaution.

Let's not miss the main point here. Training significantly increases red blood cells for oxygen transport and at the same time makes blood easier to pump because the volume of blood is greater. Both of these phenomena yield a two-way advantage to the athlete. First, his muscles receive more oxygen, more nutrition, in less time and, second, his heart and lungs accomplish their tasks with less effort. As with so many of the body changes that result from exercise, these are synergistic. In an escalating spiral, the athlete performs more easily so he trains at ever higher levels, which, in turn, pushes his tissues to adapt further, allowing him to perform even better.

6

Swimming and Walking

People ask more questions about walking and swimming than about any other exercise. Maybe it's because everybody knows how to do them, or maybe it's because they are the refuge activities of people so out of shape that every other activity looms as unpleasant.

Fat Swimmers? — an Update

She Walks, He Jogs

Fit People Think Walking Is Too Hard

Will Walking Make Me Fit?

Fat Swimmers? — an Update

My comments on swimming in *Fit or Fat?* sure raised a ruckus. You'd think I had attacked motherhood and apple pie! Angry swimmers would jump up during my lectures, challenge me to find any fat on their bodies, and declare that swimming does NOT make you fat! Actually, if you look back at what I wrote, you'll see that I never said swimming makes you fat; I only said that if you *are* fat, swimming is not the best fat-reducing exercise.

My usual flip explanation used to be, "I don't know why it's hard to lose fat with swimming. Ask a seal!" When you think about it, this answer makes sense. Mammals have a marvelous ability to adapt to their environment. Did you ever see a fat fox? Or a skinny seal? Each animal has adapted to the demands of its environment. Foxes need to trot for hours at a time, so excess fat is a burden. Seals need to search for fish in very cold water, and their extra fat provides warmth and buoyancy. Are foxes in better condition than seals because they have less fat? That's a silly question. There are fit foxes and fit, fat seals.

When I wrote *Fit or Fat?* my comments on swimming were based largely on personal observation. I had tested thousands of people for body fat and noticed that those who took up swimming for exercise seemed to have a lot of trouble reducing their total body fat. When I tested them for fitness, they showed great improvement, but their body fat stubbornly remained the same. Even Olympic-caliber swimmers tend to carry a bit more fat

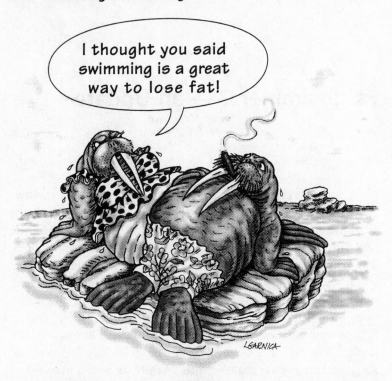

than their running counterparts. Male Olympic swimmers average 10 percent fat and females average 15 percent. That's very low fat, and their sleek bodies look great. But they are still fatter, by 4 to 5 percent, than Olympic runners.

"How can someone be more fit yet not lose fat?" I asked myself. One explanation might be food. In a recent study a group of overweight middle-aged women was divided into three exercise groups: running, bicycling, and swimming. They were told to exercise one hour a day, and they were allowed to eat as much as they wanted. After six months the runners and cyclists had lost an average of fifteen pounds. The swimmers had *gained* five pounds. The researchers speculated that the swimmers' bodies didn't want to let their fat deposits get depleted and that somehow the hypothalamus in the brain was triggered to gear up the appetite control center. "She's swimming! We'd better make her eat more so she won't lose any fat!"

Do all swimmers eat more? The ones I tested swore they didn't. "No way!" they said. "We're exercising as much as the runners and eating all those high-fiber seeds and twigs you recommend. How come the runners are losing fat and we aren't?"

Now that we have better techniques for measuring body fat, we know that the swimmers were actually losing fat from their muscles and relocating it beneath the skin where it would keep them warm and help them stay afloat. The net effect was little or no fat loss.

If you want to lose fat, don't swim!

Women, fat people, and beginning swimmers have a particularly hard time losing fat when they exercise in water. Let's look at each category.

An average woman carries more fat than an average man. You would think she'd stay warmer in water, but in fact she does not. Unless she is obese, her body cools *more* rapidly than a man's. Although fat serves as insulation, it's mainly muscle that keeps you warm in cold water, and men have more muscle than women. When you're immersed in water, the capillaries in the muscles constrict, or close up, so that warm blood can be redirected to vital organs that need the protection. The muscle then becomes an insulating shell just like fat. In fact, muscle provides 70 to 90 percent of the body's insulation in cold water, whereas fat accounts for 10 to 30 percent.

The funny thing is, even though women cool faster, it's the men who are the first to start shivering. And men warm themselves much more vigorously than women do. In other words, women are colder but don't notice it as much as men do. Their bodies don't react to it as quickly, and they don't do as much activity to warm up. This "thermal insensitivity" gives us at least three reasons why women may have a hard time burning calories when they exercise in cold water. First, they don't shiver as much. Second, they aren't as active. And finally, when they do exercise they tend to be less vigorous than men because they don't feel as cold.

The differences we see between men and women with average levels of fat become more pronounced in fatter people because thermal insensitivity to cold water increases. Fat people generally don't exercise as hard in cold water as thin people. Moreover, fat people hold on to their body heat in water. Heat loss equals calorie burning, so fat people don't use as many calories to stay warm in the water.

The third group of people who have trouble losing fat by swimming are beginners. As I've pointed out over and over, fat is lost more easily when you exercise aerobically. Beginning swimmers have a lot of problems trying to stay aerobic. They can't breathe very well, so their muscles go into oxygen deficits more often. For an *untrained* person, swimming is half aerobic and half anaerobic.

Remember also that water, because it is cooler than the body, induces constriction of the capillaries in the muscles. Although the constriction is somewhat attenuated with exercise, the capillaries still don't get as engorged as they do with activity on dry land. This means that muscles, which need lots of oxygen for aerobic work, tend to go into an anaerobic state more easily when you swim because there's less oxygen-supplying blood available.

Competitive swimmers develop a high tolerance to the lowered oxygen supply. They *want* to produce lactic acid because it's been shown that a high tolerance for lactate correlates with faster times. So anaerobic activity isn't bad; it's just that if you want the fat-burning benefits of aerobic activity, swimming may not be the best way to get them.

Beginning swimmers also need to know that resting heart rate decreases ten beats per minute in water, and maximum heart rate decreases by ten to thirty beats. The heart puts out just as much blood as in other exercises because it pumps more volume with each stroke, but more slowly. No one is certain why heart rate decreases in water, but the lower temperature and lesser pull of gravity in water may be the cause.

In any case, if you know what your exercise heart rate should be (65–80 percent of maximum) that number should be lower by at least ten beats if you swim. Here is a perfect example of why it's better to swim at the pace that is comfortable for you (see "Covert's Home Fitness Test") than to try to follow some heart rate chart. I know of one man who kept trying to swim at 80 percent of his on-land maximum heart rate and couldn't figure out why it was so exhausting. His poor muscles were having enough trouble trying to suck up oxygen from partially constricted capillaries, and he was compounding the problem by swimming at an anaerobic pace!

Elite swimmers, like other highly trained athletes, can do very intense work yet still remain aerobic. They have trained so long and so well that their muscles are capable of extracting lots of oxygen despite the metabolic restrictions mentioned earlier.

This might explain why untrained swimmers don't lose fat while trained swimmers don't get fat. Elite swimmers tend to do aerobic, fat-burning swimming; untrained swimmers do anaerobic, sugar-burning swimming.

It's a shame that it's hard to lose fat by swimming, because I think water exercise is the best thing you can do if you are fat or have arthritis or joint problems or are pregnant. It's the most injury-free sport around. Fat people who take up running hurt themselves too darn much. They're just too heavy and awkward. But how can you hurt yourself in the water? Besides, swimming is fun for the fat person. She doesn't overheat, her extra weight doesn't hinder her, she doesn't even have to know how to swim. She can do high jumps and "moon walking" in the shallow end of the pool.

Don't misinterpret what I've been saying. You *can* lose weight by swimming; you just won't lose as rapidly as if you ran or cycled. In the meantime, if you are fat, you can build fitness and agility by swimming so that, eventually, you can branch out into activities that consume more calories without risking injury.

Swimming is an excellent exercise because it is nontraumatic. You don't hear people say, "I strained my hip yesterday while swimming" or, "I wish I had been wearing my helmet when I fell down swimming." The trick is to use this exercise in the right way. Long-distance runners and cyclists do far better if they replace one or two days of their favorite sport with swimming. Then they can train at very intense levels while minimizing soreness and injuries.

Swimming and Bone Density

Swimmers' bones are less dense than the bones of any other kind of athlete. This fact has led people to the false conclusion that the antigravity properties of swimming make bones weak. Actually, studies have shown that swimming makes your bones stronger. Researchers used to think that only weight-bearing exercises increased bone density, but they now know that any exercise that tugs and pulls on tendons and ligaments, and therefore on bones, increases the deposition of calcium and phosphorus. This makes bones stronger. All the different strokes and movements in swimming certainly do a lot of joint pulling and tugging.

It's more reasonable to conclude that swimming as a sport attracts lighter-boned people. Do you ever see black people competing in swimming events? No! Black people have very heavy, dense bones; they sink like rocks in water. All their energy is used in staying afloat. It's like the question, which came first — the chicken or the egg? Swimming doesn't make bones lighter; lighter-boned people like to swim.

She Walks, He Jogs

Years ago a friend, Lea, who likes to walk rather than jog, urged me to walk with her for a week instead of doing my usual jog. Being a gallant man, I acquiesced, and we walked together for one week. At first I enjoyed it a lot. But after six days my knees began to hurt. Lea walks very fast. She is comfortable walking at a pace that's not comfortable for me. On the eighth day I finally said, "Lea, I'm sorry, but I'm going to jog for a while." It turned out that when she walked and I jogged, we stayed at almost the same pace. But I found it more comfortable to jog slowly than to walk fast.

I have horses on my farm, and that experience got me to thinking about horses. They've done all sorts of heart and lung research on two-million-dollar race horses, and one experiment particularly intrigued me. The researchers asked, "If we get a horse walking and then steadily increase the speed on the treadmill, when will the horse begin to jog or trot?" After much horsing around, they found that a given horse would switch from a walk to a trot consistently at a particular speed. Then they repeated the experiment with a rider on the horse's back. The horse would switch to a trot at a different speed, but it would always switch at that same speed as long as the rider was the same.

I'm sure you're suspicious at this point. What if they used a different horse? Yes, you're right. Each horse changes to a trot at a given speed, but the speed varies from horse to horse. It appears that switching from a walk to a trot has something to do with bones, joints, and the animal's comfort level, so different horses change from a walk to a trot at different speeds. Apparently my friend Lea's bones, joints, and knees are built in such a way that walking fast is comfortable for her, while my bones and joints are made so that walking fast is not comfortable. I prefer to jog.

> **For some people, jogging is more comfortable than walking.**

Fit People Think Walking Is Too Hard

A two-part study was done on a group of men in their mid-twenties who were fit and low in fat. In the first part they had to walk at a pace that got their heart rates to 65 percent of maximum. Then they jogged at a pace that brought their heart rates to 65 percent of maximum. This pace worked out to be approximately 4.7 miles an hour for both the walking and jogging, which is moderate for jogging but very fast for walking. In the second part of the study they had to get their heart rates to 75 percent of maximum. They achieved 75 percent by running six miles an hour, but they couldn't walk fast enough to get their heart rates that high. They finally had to walk on an inclined treadmill in order to match the running heart rate.

In both experiments these very fit men felt as if they were working harder when they were walking than when they were running, even though their heart rates were the same. It's easy to see why they felt overworked when walking. In the first experiment, when they had to walk fast enough to get their hearts to 65 percent of maximum, the pace was between twelve and thirteen minutes a mile. At that speed, regular walking feels awkward and unbalanced. Most people are more comfortable if they break into a gentle jog. In the second experiment, when the men had to walk fast enough to get to 75 percent, the treadmill had to be on an incline, which of course is more tiring than level locomotion.

My point is that fit people may find it difficult to exercise aerobically by walking. Fast walking, at aerobic intensities, is just too darn hard for them. These people may need to find routes that include some uphill sections, or they may need to wear a weighted backpack or learn race-walking techniques so they can be comfortable at faster speeds.

> **If a walker and a jogger go at the same speed and heart rate, who burns more fat?**

The question is, why does it feel easier to jog when you reach a certain speed? Part of the reason is that, as in the horse experiments discussed in the last chapter, shifting to jogging makes the joints more comfortable at a certain speed. Surprisingly, another part of the answer may have to do with calorie expenditure. Theoretically, if the distance is the same, the body should burn the same number of calories whether you walk or jog. The laws of physics tell us that it requires a certain amount of energy to cover a fixed distance. But in practice it doesn't work that way. Joggers use more energy to run three miles than walkers use to walk that distance. Running or jogging not only uses more muscles than walking, the muscles are also used more vigorously, with more heat, friction, and vertical movement (bouncing up and down).

As the speed of walking approaches that of running, the difference in calorie expenditure tends to decrease. In the study on fit young men who walked and ran at the same heart rate, running used only slightly more calories than walking. But there was a significant difference in the kind of fuel used. *A higher percentage of fat was burned during jogging than during walking.* This is the opposite of what you'd expect and seems to blow the "more fat is burned at low intensity" theory. Actually it doesn't contradict the theory at all but reinforces it.

Remember that the men felt more exhausted walking than running? That's because they were using fewer muscles when they walked, and the pace required to get to 65 percent or 75 percent of maximum heart rate tired those fewer muscles. When the men jogged, they used more muscles, so each muscle was working at lower intensity. Intensity of exercise per pound of muscle used is less in the jogger because the effort is spread out. When a muscle works at lower intensity, it burns more fat.

Keep in mind, we're talking about fit people. For them, the effort required to make walking aerobic is too intense for the number of muscles used. When a person is fat, older, or unfit, the pace required to make walking aerobic is greatly reduced.

Will Walking Make Me Fit?

In the table below I've sorted a number of exercises into categories of intensity. You can make any of these exercises harder or easier, of course, but, if allowed to go at their own pace, people tend to do them at the intensity listed. For most people running requires a lot of effort, jogging is more moderate, and their self-selected walking pace usually falls in the low-intensity range.

Intensity of Different Kinds of Exercise

High	Moderate	Low
Running	Jogging	Walking
High-impact aerobics	Low-impact aerobics	Mini-trampoline
Jumping rope	Stair climbing	
Mountain biking	Swimming	
	Rowing	
	Stationary bicycling	
	Cross-country skiing	

When young, fit people walk at a comfortable pace, the speed is usually too slow to give aerobic benefits. In other words, for young, fit people, walking isn't much of an exercise because it is simply too easy. As we get older or less fit, walking gets progressively harder and is more and more of an aerobic exercise.

You might think that younger, fitter people would make walking aerobic simply by walking faster or more vigorously, but they do not. Comfortable self-selected walking rarely exceeds 3.5 miles per hour, which just isn't fast enough to be aerobic for someone who is young and fit. If they power walk, race walk, or carry weights, the intensity changes dramatically.

If you are over sixty-five or are quite out of shape, you probably self-select a walking pace of 2–2.5 miles per hour. Even though your pace is slower, it usually is enough to be in the aerobic range. So walking does provide aerobic benefits for some people.

> **Most people self-select a walking pace that is too slow to yield aerobic benefits.**

But for almost anyone the self-selected walking pace tends to be low intensity. Even for the older or unfit person, the typical walking pace puts the heart rate in the lower part of the aerobic range.

A woman came up to me at one of my lectures to tell me that walking is more effective if you swing your arms vigorously. She went on and on about how she swung her arms vigorously when she walked. Reader, stand up right where you are and swing your arms back and forth. Then stop swinging them. Which takes more energy, getting them to swing or stopping them? I'm being a little silly here, but what I'm trying to say is that it doesn't take any effort to swing your arms. They practically swing by themselves, just as your legs almost swing by themselves when you walk. So swinging your arms does not add much intensity to walking.

Unfortunately, some readers will now conclude that walking is useless. That's NOT what I'm saying. I'm saying that because walking uses a limited amount of muscle, you have to walk a long time and do a whole lot of arm swinging before your body notices that you are exercising. Visit any hospital to see what I mean. There are people who are practically dead walking around the halls. Even after surgery you can get up and walk.

The main drawback to walking is that it takes time. A forty-minute walk at a pace that puts your heart rate in the lower end of the training zone yields results similar to a fifteen-minute jog with a heart rate in the upper end of the training zone. Those of us who don't have that much time need to find ways to increase the intensity if we want walking to be our exercise. Remember that aerobic exercise has three parameters: duration, frequency, and intensity. Of the three, intensity is the most critical; that is, fitness improves fastest when the intensity, or difficulty, of the exercise is high. For busy people it's impractical to increase the other two parameters, frequency and duration. After all, most people have only so much time to spend getting fit. Raising intensity is the easiest.

One way to make walking more intense is to carry hand weights. Heart rate speeds up five to ten beats a minute with weights, which might be just enough to put you in the training zone. Using hand weights also increases your tendency to burn fat during the exercise. Because you're using more total musculature, each muscle is being worked less intensely, which means more fat calories are used. Thus it's possible that a walker with hand weights may burn more *fat calories* than a faster walker without weights, even though *total calorie* expenditure for both walkers is about the same.

You see that the question of whether walking will get you fit depends on how fit you are to begin with. Unfit people can get into the training zone very easily by walking. As your fitness improves you need to raise the intensity by walking faster and faster or carrying more weight or finding uphill routes. I know one really fit guy who doesn't run because it bothers his knees, so he walks uphill for five miles every day — carrying his golden retriever on his back! I'm kidding, of course, but you get the point. If you want to get fit by walking, you have to do a lot of it or alter it in some way to make it more intense.

If you think my analysis implies that walking is useless, join me this weekend for a six-hour stroll above timberline on Mount Hood. It will be gentle, safe, aerobic, pleasant, and one hell of an aerobic conditioner. In a way, walking is the perfect exercise because it requires no equipment and no instruction. It's a natural part of so many favorite pastimes like golf, hiking, archery, some forms of fishing, and hunting that it fits easily into most lifestyles. Don't take my analysis as a downer. The gentleness of walking is its good point.

7

Before Exercise — and After

Warming Up Before Exercise

During exercise the temperature inside muscle gradually rises, which dramatically changes the muscle's ability to use the oxygen and fuel delivered by the blood. When blood passes through cold muscles, oxygen can't detach itself from its hemoglobin very easily. It's as if the oxygen says, "It's too cold in there. I'm staying right here in the blood with my hemoglobin buddy." As muscle temperature rises, oxygen breaks away from the hemoglobin more rapidly and more completely. If you plunge into an activity without warming up, your "cold" muscles are, in effect, oxygen-starved for the first few minutes.

You've probably experienced this phenomenon although you may not have understood it. There have been days when you haven't had time to warm up, and the first ten minutes of jogging, even though you were going at your usual pace, got you out of breath. Essentially, you were jogging anaerobically because your muscles lacked oxygen. Your body hadn't warmed up enough for oxygen to easily separate from hemoglobin. Later on, you were comfortable running at the same speed that initially got you breathless. Lesson learned! Start your run at a slower speed until the muscles are warmed so that oxygen can easily be released from the hemoglobin.

Inside the muscle cells, the rise in temperature accelerates the activity of all those enzymes we've talked about. Fats and sugars are broken down more rapidly, which means that ATP is produced more quickly and less lactic acid accumulates.

Because warm muscles are more elastic, they are less susceptible to injury. Warmer temperatures produce a fluidlike stretch that allows greater range of motion. Cold muscles don't absorb shock or impact as well and don't stretch as well so they get injured more readily.

Muscles aren't the only beneficiaries of warming up. Higher temperatures improve the function of the nervous system, meaning that messages are carried more rapidly to and from the brain or spinal cord. Whether you're an elite athlete needing to make split-second decisions or a twelve-minute-mile jogger whose only problem is avoiding a rock in your path, a warmed-up nervous system helps you to coordinate intricate movements.

> **If you warm up first, you'll burn more fat.**

The capillaries that weave around the muscles also respond to the warmer temperature by dilating. This brings more oxygen to the muscles and helps in the removal of waste products such as carbon dioxide and lactic acid.

The heart also benefits from warming up. Studies have shown heart irregularities in people who exercise without warming up. In one experiment, when healthy men exercised vigorously on a treadmill for ten to fifteen seconds with no prior warm-up, electrocardiogram readings showed abnormal changes in 70 percent of them. No correlation could be found with age or fitness; that is, young fit men showed as many abnormalities as older or unfit ones. When the test was repeated after a warm-up, the irregular findings either completely disappeared or were greatly diminished.

Perhaps most important, warmed muscles burn fat more readily than cold muscles. The implications of this go deeper than you might think. Fat is released during stress. The stress of sudden, intense exercise causes a deluge of fatty acids into the bloodstream. If you start your exercise at full speed, your cold muscles can't use the fatty acids, and they end up in places where they aren't wanted, such as the lining of your arteries.

In summary, a warmed-up body

- Enhances vasodilation so that more blood is delivered to the muscles
- Allows oxygen in the blood to detach from the hemoglobin more easily
- Speeds up the breakdown of glucose and fatty acids
- Makes muscles more elastic, less susceptible to injury
- Improves coordination
- Reduces heart irregularities associated with sudden exercise
- Burns fat more easily

How to Warm Up

Some people, hearing that warming up is important, try the most bizarre things. They take hot baths, saunas, heating pads, or massage, none of which work because they raise only the body's *surface* temperature. True, the muscles are warmed, but alterations in chemical, neural, and cellular function are dependent on changes in deep core temperature, which isn't affected much by these external heat sources. If you spend too much time in a sauna, your internal heat does, in fact, build up — but this systemic heat is not the specific deep muscle heat we want and actually decreases your level of performance.

The most widely used warm-up techniques are jogging, calisthenics, rope jumping, and stationary bicycling. All work well to elevate deep muscle temperature and rev up the physiological changes we've talked about. A warm-up can be just a slow version of the upcoming exercise. Walk before jogging. Jog before running. Bicycle, row, or aerobic-dance at a slower pace than the actual exercise.

To warm up a specific muscle, do the same movements — but less intensely — that you do during the actual event. It's a walk-through rehearsal of what's to come. For instance, a tennis player practices her swing more slowly and a baseball pitcher throws more gently.

For sports you may need to do both overall *and* specific warm-ups. Weightlifters, for example, should warm up the entire body first. A jog or fast walk to the weightlifting facility, if it's not far away, is a good general warm-up. If this isn't con-

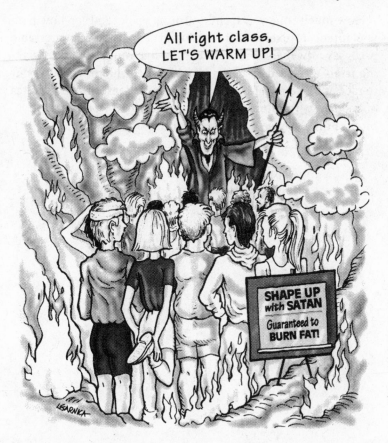

venient, use a stationary bicycle, stair climber, or treadmill once you're there. Eight to twelve minutes should be enough time for a general warm-up prior to weightlifting. Then warm up specific muscles by using lighter weights for the first few repetitions.

It isn't practical to measure your muscle temperature, so use heart rate and breathing as guidelines. Warm up at a pace that gets your heart beating at 50–60 percent of your maximum (compared to 65–80 percent of MHR during actual exercise). You should be breathing harder than normal but not as hard as during the actual exercise.

How much time you spend warming up depends on how hard you intend to exercise. If you jog at a relatively comfortable pace, say a twelve-minute mile, then five minutes of fast walking is all you need to warm up. An elite athlete who is about to race at a five-minute-mile pace needs at least fifteen minutes of moderate running to warm up. In other words, the more intense the exercise, the longer you need to warm up.

> **A good warm-up can be simply a slower version of the upcoming exercise.**

Delayed Muscle Soreness

When a muscle is subjected to an intense unfamiliar exercise, it usually gets delayed muscle soreness — DMS. Even a weight-lifter's muscle that is used to a specific exercise gets DMS when extra "unfamiliar" weight is added. I'm not talking about the lactic acid pain that occurs immediately with exercise. I'm talking about that stiff, tender feeling that comes on one or two days after exercise and makes your muscles ache for a day or two.

DMS is a peculiar pain phenomenon in that it doesn't hurt at the time of injury. Normally, if you injure yourself, say by putting your hand on a hot stove, it hurts right away. But with DMS, the pain occurs twenty-four hours after the activity. If your body didn't like what was happening to it, why didn't it hurt during the activity?

You say, "Well, maybe it hurts the next day as a sort of protection. Perhaps the delayed pain prevents you from exercising again, thereby protecting the muscles from further injury." This sounds plausible except that the best way to alleviate DMS is to do a milder version of the same exercise that brought on the pain in the first place!

Here's another peculiar thing about DMS. Usually, an injury hurts a lot at first and gradually lessens as the injured area heals. But DMS does just the opposite. You don't hurt at all at first, but the pain gets worse as the muscle heals. And muscle strength returns before the pain goes away. Tests have shown that in the period between exercise and the onset of DMS, your muscles can't exert as much force. Yet muscle force returns to normal about twenty-four hours after the exercise — just when the pain sensation has reached maximum intensity!

> **Next-day muscle pain is completely different from other kinds of body pain.**

No one really knows what causes DMS. Some researchers say it's nothing more than small tears in the muscle tissue, while others blame free radicals, high muscle temperatures, or a change in acidity of the fluids in the muscles. Whatever the cause, once a muscle fiber cell is injured, it goes on an automatic, built-in self-destruction program. First, the walls of the cell become more permeable, and substances leak out that shouldn't, such as enzymes and proteins, which then show up in the urine. And substances leak into the cell that shouldn't, one of which is calcium. Normally there is more calcium outside the muscle cell than inside, but when the cell starts leaking, more calcium shows up inside. The calcium activates a certain protein-dissolving enzyme that attacks and destroys the cell membrane. Now there's a real mess in the muscles.

When the membrane is destroyed, the innards of the cell spill out. This attracts water to dilute the concentration, as well as certain white blood cells called macrophages, the "garbage collectors" of the immune system. They find all the dead and dying cells and cry, "Yo! Free food! Let's eat!" The macrophages rush in to consume the dead cellular debris. Like sharks in a feeding frenzy, they're too impatient to wait for the dying cells to die, so they produce membrane-dissolving enzymes of their own to speed up the process.

This combination of dying cells, marauding macrophages, spilled enzymes, and water builds and builds until, about twenty-four hours after the exercise, nerve endings in the area begin to get irritated. Normally, these nerve endings, called group IV fibers, are easygoing guys. They have a high tolerance for noxious stimuli, but after twenty-four hours they've had it. They start transmitting a dull, diffuse pain, and you start feeling sore.

Thankfully, the damage is not permanent. If you could look through a microscope at a piece of muscle during DMS, you'd see new fiber being made in the midst of all that destruction. Muscle tissue after a bout of DMS is actually more resistant to future injury and repairs faster when injured. Considering the number of episodes of DMS athletes experience during their careers, it's a good thing the long-term effects are positive.

How to Prevent Sore Muscles

Training provides protection from delayed muscle soreness. The more trained muscles you have, the fewer episodes of DMS you'll experience. With training, as the saying goes, "A little bit goes a long way." A little bit of stress to a muscle provides up to six weeks of protection against DMS from a larger stress to the same muscle.

For example, a group of women lifted a weight seventy times with one arm. Then they lifted the same weight with the other arm twenty-four times. As expected, the muscles in the arm that did seventy lifts developed severe DMS, while the muscles in the arm that did twenty-four lifts got mild DMS. Two weeks later the women did seventy lifts with the arm that had previously done twenty-four. They expected to get the debilitating soreness they had earlier gotten from doing seventy repetitions but were surprised that the symptoms were again mild. The twenty-four initial lifts apparently ameliorated the effects of the seventy subsequent contractions.

In other words, a relatively small injury to muscle causes it to adapt, becoming more resistant to future damage. In practical terms, you can do short bouts of downhill running if you know that your next race has a long stretch of downhill. Before next winter's cross-country ski trip, you can work out on a cross-country ski machine.

When you do get DMS, even though it's encouraging to know that the muscle is repairing and actually getting more resistant to injury, you're still stuck with the pain. The best way to stop it is to do a gentler version of the exercise that initiated it. No one knows why this works. Some say adhesions from the injury are broken by repeating the exercise. Other researchers think that exercise may stimulate the release of endorphins, the body's natural painkillers, which then dampen the symptoms of DMS.

> **"Should I exercise when my muscles are sore?"**

The simplest and most likely explanation is that exercise increases activity in the large nerve fibers, which interfere with, or override, the pain sensations. The large nerve fibers are mainly concerned with touch and temperature. When they are stimulated, they override pain sensations caused by smaller nerve fibers. This is known as a "gating" mechanism; the activity of one set of nerve fibers "closes the gate" or shuts out signals from another set of fibers. When a painful stimulus occurs — say you step on a sharp object — the smaller pain fibers are activated. These overcome the inhibition of the large fibers so that your foot can tell the brain, "Hey! I'm hurt!" Your immediate reaction is to rub your foot. Rubbing increases the touch sensation, which activates the large nerve fibers. This "closes the gate" or modulates the activity of the small pain fibers. So rubbing a sore foot — or a sore muscle — won't make it better, but it will make it hurt less. Doing the same exercise to relieve DMS probably produces heat and friction in the sore muscles, which triggers the large nerve fibers to override the pain sensations of the smaller fibers.

The large nerve fibers can also be activated by heat or massage. There are all kinds of liniments and ointments for muscle soreness. While it is doubtful that medications or massage actually speed up the repair process, the rubbing and the heat produced activate the large nerve fibers to provide temporary relief from pain.

The Lowdown on Rubdowns

I never had a massage until I was about fifty-two years old. Even though I did lots of sports and had been treated for many injuries, I hadn't tried the massage experience. Wow, what a neat sensation! I felt pampered, cared for, rich, free, and relaxed. "This is good for me," I said to myself. "Anything that makes me feel this good has *got* to be good for me."

At the time I didn't think about practical questions, such as will I sleep better? Will my muscles recuperate from today's exercise faster? Will I compete better tomorrow? I just soaked it up, enjoyed it, and felt like a king.

As I was preparing to leave, I expressed my enthusiasm to the masseuse. She told me that massage speeds the healing of sore muscles by getting rid of toxins. She said it oxygenates muscles and improves exercise performance. Naturally my curiosity was aroused. I left there believing in her magical prowess for making me *feel* better. But I also left eager to read some research on massage. Could her claims be true?

Somehow the myth has evolved that our muscles are filled with "toxins" that can be squeezed out with massage. But if I ask, "What kinds of toxins are there in muscles?" I usually get a blank look. I'm not saying there aren't noxious products that accumulate in overworked muscles, such as those associated with DMS. I'm just annoyed that "toxin" has become such a catchall scare word lately. "We need to get a massage to get rid of toxins." "We need to fast to get rid of toxins." "We need to take castor oil to get rid of toxins." Come on, guys! Give it a break. Read up on your physiology before you continue to rattle off such nonsense.

Regardless of what the toxins are, does massage speed up the elimination of waste products from damaged muscle tissue? Researchers designed an experiment to answer that question. Elite male cyclists cycled a hundred miles a day for four days. At the end of each day, half of the men received a massage and the other half had a microwave tissue heating treatment. Actually, the second group *thought* they were getting a microwave treatment, but the machine was inactivated, so they were, in effect, a placebo group; they were getting no therapy at all.

> **"Does massage help eliminate toxins from sore muscles?"**

You can bet that the massage group was happier and probably felt better, but did they eliminate more "toxins"? The researchers tested every conceivable thing. They tested for the breakdown products of muscle enzymes and liver enzymes, including creatine kinase, lactate dehydrogenase, creatinine, aspartate aminopeptidase, alanine aminotransferase, and gamma glutamyl transpeptidase. They tested blood and they tested urine. They looked at electrolytes and hormones. And guess what they found? Absolutely no difference between the two groups! To make sure there wasn't some weird coincidence, the experiment was repeated in three weeks, this time switching the groups. The results were the same.

In other words, those chemicals — toxins, if you wish — that appear in the body and in muscle after strenuous exercise are not removed, transported, or "detoxified" differently if you get a massage.

Companion to the claim that massage squeezes toxins out of the muscles is the assertion that it also gets more oxygen and nutrients *into* the muscles by increasing blood flow. But blood flow to parts of the body is carefully regulated; it increases in specific areas only through metabolic demand. If a tissue needs more oxygen or fuel, arterioles open up to deliver more blood to meet the demand. In tissues at rest, blood supply is limited.

A vigorous massage gives a rosy glow and warm feeling to the skin, indicating that the capillaries beneath the skin surface have been stimulated to open up. But the effect is only temporary. The muscles in the area aren't working and therefore don't need the extra blood. As soon as the massage is over, the capillaries close up, and the muscles never partake of their temporary oxygen feast.

An even sillier claim — one few therapists make, thank God — is that massage gets rid of body fat. Fat can ONLY be used, burned, and eliminated by muscles. It can't be rubbed off or sweated off or pounded off. Even the idea that massage loosens up fat so that it is burned more easily is ludicrous. Should you somehow be able to release fat from fat pads via massage (which you can't), what would happen to it? It would travel to the muscle and ask, "Do you want me?" And the muscles would reply, "Go away, fatty. We don't need you right now. We're getting massaged." The only one who loses fat during a massage is the massager!

Another "big benefit" of massage, advocates say, is that it improves performance. But the hundred-mile-a-day cycling study couldn't find any difference. In fact, some of the placebo group outperformed the massage group. The question then arises, "Does massage make you feel better so that you're psychologically prepared to perform better?" To test this, both groups took a Profile of Mood States questionnaire each night after their massage or fake microwave treatment. Here there *was* a difference. The massage group got much higher positive ratings. Whether the massage itself elevated their mood or whether they were happier just because someone was caring for them (the "hands-on," or touching response), researchers couldn't tell. But by the next morning, when the cyclists knew they had another grueling one hundred miles ahead of them, both groups scored equally low on the mood scale.

Some massage therapists take a different tack concerning performance. They say that massage loosens muscles, which helps prevent injury. With less down time from injury, more time can be spent improving performance. It may be true that massage loosens muscles, but does it work any better than the standard warming-up and stretching techniques used by athletes? Probably not. The best way to raise muscle temperature is by exercising the muscle. Massage may have a loosening effect, but it does not eliminate the need to actively warm up the muscle. The same goes for the claim that massage breaks up adhesions formed when muscles are injured. It probably does break up adhesions, but no more effectively than sensible stretching.

One claim that might have some merit is that massage relaxes muscles. A characteristic of fatigued muscle is that it can't relax. Have you noticed after a long, strenuous hike how hard it is to keep your feet and legs still? You have to flex your muscles every now and then to help them relax. Massage probably does the same thing.

Another benefit of massage is that it relieves muscle soreness. Massaging tender muscles activates the large touch and sensation nerve fibers, which tend to override the impulses sent out by the smaller pain fibers, so you don't feel as sore (see "Delayed Muscle Soreness"). So while massage may not be able to get rid of the cause of sore muscles, it does alleviate the pain associated with them. This relief from pain allows you to use the muscle more freely, which speeds the healing process.

Massage doesn't speed up the removal of waste products or fat, it doesn't add more oxygen or nutrients, and it doesn't appreciably affect performance. Does that mean it's useless? Certainly not! Massage feels wonderful. We all know that many animals enjoy being stroked, actively seeking it from other animals or from humans whenever possible. It's a funny human quirk that whenever something is uncomfortable, we figure it must be good for us — the no-pain, no-gain syndrome. But when something feels great, we think we have to come up with all sorts of scientific reasons for why we need it. All I've been trying to point out is that the current crop of "scientific" benefits of massage either haven't been substantiated or haven't been shown to be better than what the body ordinarily does for itself.

It may turn out that massage does nothing more than have a pleasant effect on sensory nerves, which produces a feeling of well-being. Or maybe there's still some undiscovered reason why it's good for us. Perhaps in a few years we will have solid evidence that massage has specific, measurable physical effects. In the meantime, enjoy it!

8

Measuring Your Own Fat and Fitness

*You can spend lots of dollars at fancy clinics
getting fancy tests, but nothing beats
self-measurement. Home tests let you set
your own goals — the best motivation
for high achievement.*

Covert's Home Fitness Test

The Home Body-Fat Test

Potbellies and Thunder Thighs

The Waist-to-Hip-Ratio Test

Are Home Tests Really Useful?

Covert's Home Fitness Test

I'm going to describe a home fitness test that costs nothing, is self-administered, and doesn't hurt. In a sense, "my test" isn't mine at all because joggers use it already. When those who jog for fitness (not competition runners) discuss their daily jog, it is common to hear them discuss their "pace." They are referring to the average number of minutes it takes them to jog a mile. Some of them jog two miles and some seven miles. Some jog once a week, others every day. Despite the disparity in their routines, the expression "pace" provides common ground for discussion.

Pace, or minutes per mile, does not imply maximum. It is not at all the same as asking, "How fast can you run a mile?" Quite the opposite. It means, "How fast can you run a mile without discomfort *and do the same tomorrow and again the next day?*" This last clause eliminates one of the first objections to using the "pace" concept as the basis for my test. The objection would be that two people might claim the same pace, for example, a nine-minute mile, and therefore the same level of fitness, but one does it at 85 percent of maximum heart rate while the other is only at 70 percent. Obviously they are not equally fit. But is their pace really the same? Among those who jog almost every day, the routine minutes per mile becomes just that — routine. Their pace is, in fact, a consistently reliable indicator of their fitness. The person who ran a nine-minute mile at 85 percent of MHR cannot repeat that day after day — it is not his routine pace.

I want everyone, including those who are overweight, those who have had a heart attack, and all of you average out-of-shape types, to establish your minutes-per-mile "pace," your own aerobic, comfortable, repeatable, and consistent pace. That's my entire fitness test — DETERMINE YOUR PACE. Find out how fast you can cover a mile comfortably, repeatedly, and consistently. I don't care if you run, jog, or walk. If you're too fat or out of shape to even walk, lie down and roll! For one week, do that mile every day at a speed that feels comfortable. Can you talk haltingly? Are you breathing deeply but not panting? By the end of the week you should know your pace. You should know how many minutes it takes you to go one mile comfortably. Your pace may be a five-minute run if you're very fit or a twenty-minute walk if you're out of shape.

If you're too fat or out of shape to walk, lie down and roll!

An Olympic runner can sprint one four-minute mile, can race consecutive five-minute miles, and can talk conversationally at a six-minute-mile aerobic pace. That runner could confuse the issue by claiming a five-minute pace or, worse, a four-minute pace. We are not interested in his sprint time; we want to know his steady aerobic pace, which is six minutes.

You will notice that I haven't mentioned taking your pulse, that is, your heart rate. It doesn't matter if your heart rate is 20 or 2,000 if you are comfortable and can repeat the exercise comfortably tomorrow. As I've emphasized, the heart rate charts on the walls of gyms or in books were devised for the "average" person, and you may not be average at all. If you don't know your maximum heart rate, you can't rely on the formula 220 − age = MHR, which is only an approximation anyway.

If you really want to match your pace to your heart rate, I urge you to determine for yourself your correct aerobic pace. If

I were helping you, I would have you walk on a treadmill with a heart rate monitor strapped around your chest. Then I would gradually increase the speed of the treadmill while I carefully noted your breathing. When you reached the point where you were breathing deeply, but not panting, and were still able to talk to me, haltingly, not fluently, I would record the pulse rate indicated on the monitor as your target aerobic heart rate.

We would have to repeat the procedure over several days and average the results before I would trust the conclusion. People who do laboratory treadmill testing believe that their skills can provide accurate aerobic heart rate zones for individuals even though they test them only once. I do not agree. Testing a person once or even twice with the best of machinery cannot match the accuracy of everyday experience.

It will be difficult for some people to give up the idea of taking a pulse and replace it with the pace concept. Your pace will inevitably be somewhere in the middle of your training zone, 65–80 percent of maximum heart rate range, which is considered aerobic by me, *Fit or Fat?* and thousands of other people in the field. The concept of training zone is still valid, but pace is an exact number within that range.

Some may criticize the pace concept on the grounds that it depends too much on personal motivation and sensation, but again I will emphasize that among people who jog, pace is incredibly accurate. It's exactly the comfort zone of an individual, and no formula or laboratory can do better. Obviously, if you have no running history and you try to determine your pace in a single day, you've missed the point.

I want *everyone* to do my fitness test. If you are very fit but don't like running or jogging, do the test anyway. If you are superfat and intimidated by runners, do the test anyway. It will be a boon to the fitness movement when everyone talks about his pace, even those who do not routinely jog. If a stranger told you on the phone that he weighed 170 pounds, you might not think much about it. But if that stranger turned out to be a deep-voiced five-foot-one woman, you *would* think about it.

Similarly, if a stranger on the telephone told you his pace was ten, you would not be impressed. But if that stranger turned out to be ninety-eight years old, it would be remarkable.

When people become familiar with the pace concept, and each person is observant of fluctuations in his own pace, we will be able to talk about health in a whole new way. People will say things like:

"I'm usually a ten, but I had a wicked cold last month and I'm down to an eleven."

"I plateaued at eleven point five for nearly a year. Couldn't seem to improve until my divorce finalized, then I shot up to a nine."

"I can't believe it! I've gone from an eleven to a ten in two weeks just by eating less fat."

The Home Body-Fat Test

There are many ways to measure body fat at home; I recommend the skin caliper method because of its practicality. The calipers, available from several companies, are made of plastic and usually sell for less than twelve dollars, so most people can afford to buy them. And anyone can learn how to use them. The skin caliper method is based on a simple principle, that the thickness of the fat just under your skin is a fair representation of the amount of fat elsewhere in your body. Men doubt the test's accuracy because their deep belly fat is so remote from a pinch of skin on the back of the arm. But in repeated comparisons of body fat done by the water tank method (considered the most accurate) and the skin caliper method, the calipers have been found quite useful. As men's bellies get fatter, their skin also gets fatter; that is, a thin, almost invisible layer of fat develops under the skin in direct proportion to the increase of fat inside the abdomen.

Women also find it hard to believe that a pinch of skin under their wing bone or on the back of their arm could possibly reflect the fat in their buttocks and legs. They are so aware of fat in those typical female places that they don't notice subtle fat changes in the skin over their biceps. Testing body fat by pinching the skin at three or four sites on a woman's upper body almost always produces the remark, "You obviously don't know where my fat is." In fact, we do know!

Of course, skin fat is not uniform over the whole body. The skin over the elbows usually remains quite thin even in very

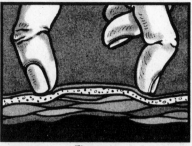

Figure a

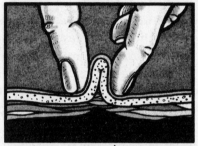

Figure b

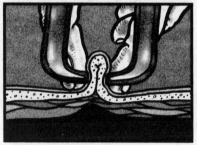

Figure c

fat people. Skin on the palms of the hands and soles of the feet also tends to remain almost fat free. But other areas get fat quite easily and four of them have become the standard pinch sites. By adding together the skin thicknesses from those four sites, we get a fair representation of total body fat.

1. Front of the arm over the biceps.
2. Back of the arm over the triceps.

3. On the back, just under the scapula or wing bone.
4. At the waist just above the hipbone.

Figures a, b, and c illustrate the basic skin-fold measurement technique. The very thin outer layer represents the skin itself. Fat is the next layer, just under the skin and attached to it. By pinching a fold of skin as shown, you are actually measuring a fold of skin and a fold of fat together. To make the measurement, you pull the skin and its attached fat away from the underlying muscle. Notice that the fingers continue to hold the skin folded while the measurement is taken. The "pinch" actually measures two thicknesses of skin and two layers of underlying fat.

The calipers are almost always calibrated in millimeters (mm.); one millimeter is approximately the thickness of a pencil lead. In a young, very fit boy, a pinch of skin on the front of the biceps may be as thin as 3 mm., about the same as taking a pinch of his shirt. A pinch of skin on the back of his arm over the triceps would be at least 5 mm. even if he was very low in fat. In other words, it's natural to have a little more fat on the back of the arm than on the front. That boy's father is probably a little fatter, so the back of his arm might have a 12-mm. skin-fold thickness. Looking at the table on page 183, you can see that measuring skin-fold thickness on the back of the arm gives an approximation of total body fat. The boy would be 8 percent fat while his father would be around 25 percent.

If skin-fold testing at just this one place gives a reasonable indication of body fat, obviously we could get more accuracy by testing a number of sites. There are clinics where no less than ten sites are measured in an effort at accuracy. I believe that using the four sites I listed earlier is good enough.

If you look at the tables on pages 185 and 186, you will notice that when the women's numbers are compared to the men's, it appears that women are getting a raw deal. Take a forty-year-old man and a forty-year-old woman, for example. If the sum of the woman's pinches adds up to 30 mm., she is 23 percent fat, but

Percentage of Body Fat in Women (Using One Location)

Back of arm skin-fold thickness (mm.)	AGE		
	15–29	*30–49*	*50+*
4	10.5	11.0	12.5
5	11.0	14.0	16.0
6	13.0	16.0	18.0
7	15.0	18.5	20.5
8	17.0	20.0	22.5
9	19.0	22.0	24.5
10	20.0	23.0	26.0
11	21.5	24.5	27.5
12	23.0	25.5	29.0
13	24.0	27.0	30.0
14	25.0	28.0	31.0
15	26.0	29.0	32.0
16	27.0	30.0	33.5
17	27.5	30.5	34.0
18	28.5	31.0	35.0
19	29.0	32.0	36.0
20	30.0	33.0	37.0
22	31.5	34.0	38.0
24	32.5	35.5	39.5
26	34.0	36.5	41.0
28	35.0	37.5	42.0
30	36.0	38.5	43.0
32	37.0	39.5	44.5
34	38.0	40.5	45.0
36	38.5	41.0	46.0
38	39.5	42.0	47.0
40	40.0	43.0	48.0
45	42.0	44.5	50.0
50	43.5	46.0	52.0
55	45.0	47.5	53.5
60	46.5	49.0	55.0
65	47.5	50.0	56.5
70	48.5	51.0	57.5
75	50.0	52.0	58.5
80	51.0	53.0	60.0

Percentage of Body Fat in Men
(Using One Location)

Back of arm skin-fold thickness (mm.)	AGE		
	_15–29_	_30–49_	_50+_
3	5.0	11.0	12.0
4	6.5	14.5	15.5
5	8.0	16.5	18.5
6	11.0	18.5	21.0
7	12.5	20.0	23.0
8	14.0	21.5	24.5
9	15.0	22.5	26.0
10	16.0	23.5	27.5
11	17.5	24.5	29.0
12	18.5	25.0	30.0
13	19.0	26.0	31.0
14	20.0	27.0	32.0
15	21.0	27.5	33.0
16	21.5	28.0	34.0
17	22.0	28.5	34.5
18	23.0	29.0	35.5
19	23.5	30.0	36.0
20	24.0	30.5	37.0
22	25.0	31.0	38.0
24	26.0	32.0	39.5
26	27.0	33.0	40.5
28	28.0	33.5	41.5
30	29.0	34.0	42.5
32	29.5	35.0	43.5
34	30.5	35.5	44.5
36	31.0	36.0	45.0
38	31.5	36.5	46.0
40	32.0	37.0	46.5
45	33.5	38.5	48.5
50	35.0	39.5	50.0
55	36.0	40.5	51.5
60	37.0	41.5	52.5
65	38.0	42.0	53.5
70	39.0	43.0	55.0
75	39.5	43.5	56.0
80	40.5	44.5	57.0

if the man has 30 mm. he is only 17 percent fat. That doesn't seem fair. However, 15 percent fat is considered ideal for men and 22 percent ideal for women. Women are expected to have more fat than men, and therefore the charts include an extra 7–8 percent obligatory fat for women. Both the man and the woman in the example are only one to two percent above their optimum.

Notice also that as you get older, the same measurement represents more fat; it's assumed that as they get older, people are getting fatter underneath where it can't be seen, even if their skin fat hasn't thickened appreciably.

**The cheapo body-fat pincher devices
are the wave of the future.**

There are dozens of calipers on the market, too many for me to list. They're advertised in most sports and fitness magazines. A set of instructions is included, along with charts similar to the ones shown here. Some manufacturers mistakenly add another chart relating body fat to fitness. They make the assumption that people low in fat are high in fitness. DO NOT be suckered into this kind of foolishness; there are very low-fat, anorexic women who are not fit at all. Conversely, there are extremely fit athletic people who are fat because they overeat. DO NOT assume that low fat means high fitness — or vice versa.

I want to make a really strong case for these pincher devices. I believe they're the wave of the future. People think calipers aren't accurate because they're cheap, but this little cheapo method can give you some pretty solid information. You don't have to know exactly to the tenth what percentage of your body is fat. If you know it within 3 or 4 percent, you have a baseline. By testing yourself routinely every couple of months, you'll see whether your body fat goes up or down. When your body weight goes up by two pounds, it could be fat — or it could be muscle.

Percentage of Body Fat in Women
(Using Four Locations)

Sum of skin folds (mm.)	AGE		
	15–29	30–49	50+
14	9.0	14.0	17.0
15	10.5	15.0	18.0
16	11.0	15.5	18.5
18	12.5	17.0	20.0
20	14.0	18.5	21.5
25	16.5	20.0	24.0
30	19.5	23.0	26.5
35	21.5	25.0	28.5
40	23.0	26.5	30.0
45	25.0	28.0	32.0
50	26.5	29.5	33.0
55	28.0	30.5	34.5
60	29.0	32.0	35.5
65	30.0	33.0	36.5
70	31.0	34.0	37.5
75	32.0	34.5	38.5
80	33.0	35.5	39.5
85	34.0	36.0	40.0
90	35.0	37.0	41.0
95	35.5	38.0	42.0
100	36.5	38.5	42.5
105	37.0	39.0	43.0
110	37.5	39.5	44.0
115	38.0	40.0	44.5
120	39.0	41.0	45.0
125	39.5	41.5	45.5
130	40.0	42.0	46.0
135	40.5	42.5	46.5
140	41.0	43.0	47.0
150	42.0	44.0	48.0
160	43.0	44.5	49.0
170	44.5	45.5	50.0
180	45.0	46.0	51.0
190	46.0	47.0	52.0
200	46.5	47.5	52.5

Percentage of Body Fat in Men
(Using Four Locations)

Sum of skin folds (mm.)	AGE		
	15–29	*30–49*	*50+*
20	8.0	12.0	12.5
22	9.0	13.0	14.0
24	10.0	14.0	15.0
26	11.0	15.0	16.0
28	12.0	16.0	17.5
30	13.0	17.0	18.5
35	14.5	18.5	21.0
40	16.0	20.0	23.0
45	17.5	22.0	24.5
50	19.0	23.0	26.0
55	20.0	24.0	27.5
60	21.0	25.0	29.0
65	22.0	26.0	30.0
70	23.0	27.0	31.5
75	24.0	28.0	32.5
80	24.5	28.5	33.5
85	25.5	29.5	34.5
90	26.0	30.0	35.5
95	27.0	31.0	36.5
100	27.5	31.5	37.0
105	28.0	32.0	38.0
110	29.0	33.0	39.0
115	29.5	33.5	39.5
120	30.0	34.0	40.0
125	30.5	34.5	40.5
130	31.0	35.0	41.5
135	31.5	35.5	42.0
140	32.0	36.0	43.0
150	33.0	37.0	44.0
160	33.5	37.5	45.0
170	34.0	38.5	46.0
180	35.0	39.0	47.0
190	36.0	40.0	48.0
200	36.5	40.5	49.0

Using a pincher along with your bathroom scale, you can tell which it is. In other words, if your weight goes up two pounds, but your body-fat measurement indicates no change since the last time, you can say, "Whoopee! My body fat hasn't gone up. Maybe my muscle's increased!" It's also possible that the extra weight is just water, but at least you know it isn't fat. People who claim the caliper "can't be accurate" will eventually, when everyone has one, be hosting neighborhood "pinching" parties.

Get some kind of home body-fat kit, use it, and don't quibble about its accuracy. The calipers are very good tracking devices.

Potbellies and Thunder Thighs

The next chapter describes still another way of testing body fat, but it measures the difference between male and female fat, which I need to discuss before I go to the test itself.

Men do constant battle with their bellies. Eat too much one day, and there it is the next, jutting out for all to see. Eat it today, wear it tomorrow. However, when men diet or exercise, they lose their belly fat almost as easily as they gain it. It's a lot harder for women to get rid of thigh fat. Actually, it's more correct to say that male-type fat is easier to shed than female-type fat.

Even if women are careful about their diet, exercise religiously, and look fit and trim, their thighs stubbornly hold their fat. Echoing Professor Higgins in *My Fair Lady*, they wail, "Why can't my legs be more like a man's?"

I once tested a man who came out 25 percent fat (15 percent is considered healthy). He refused to believe his results. "How can you call me fat?" he indignantly asked while pounding on his skinny thighs. "My legs are as hard as rocks!" As he spoke, about thirty pounds of lard on his abdomen were quivering in shock-wave response to each blow to his leg.

Men's potbelly fat is NOT the same as "love handle" fat. I'm referring to the deep abdominal fat that causes overall rounding and tautness of the abdomen. "Love handle" fat is subcutaneous, just beneath the skin surface. You can grab it and jiggle it. The bulk of abdominal fat is under the abdominal muscles surrounding the intestines, making it hard to grab.

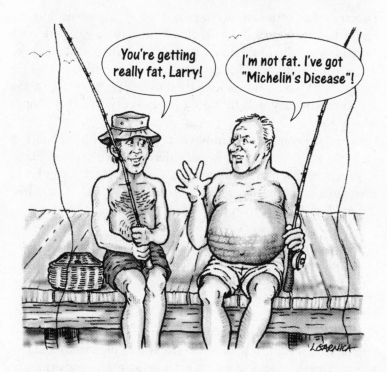

Fat distribution is almost wholly determined by genetics and sex hormones. If you are male, your fat deposits are likely to be in the typical male places. When men or women have fat in places not usually associated with their sex, it's usually because they have a little more of the opposite sex's hormones. Women with skinny legs and fatter abdomens may have additional male characteristics, such as facial or chest hair, deeper voices, or a tendency to "muscle up." Blood tests on these women show higher amounts of male sex hormones.

Classic female thigh fat has chemical characteristics that are quite different from those of male belly fat. Ordinarily, fat cells have two enzymes; one assists in fat deposition and storage while the other assists in fat release. In thigh fat, the two enzymes are quite inactive. Women think their thigh fat builds up quickly, but it does not. It builds up very slowly, starting at puberty when estrogen increases and when women usually exercise less than they did as children. Imagine a gas tank on a car with a gas filler tube about the size of a pencil. It would take a long time to fill. Imagine gas leaving the tank through another tiny tube. It would take a long time to empty. Women's thighs are like that; they will fill up with fat slowly, but they empty slowly too.

Should women starve themselves to slim their thighs? No! The body has a good reason for keeping that fat! That's why it's hard to get rid of. It's normal for women to store a little extra fat in their thighs, and using extreme methods to get rid of it is like saying, "I'm smarter than God."

> **If you want skinny legs,
> breast-feed!**

The fat depots in women's thighs and buttocks are activated only during specific female stress situations, pregnancy and lactation. The hormones of pregnancy cause the fat-depositing enzymes to be more active. Pregnant women sadly attest to this fact as they watch their thighs get fatter. But then, once the baby is born and breast-feeding commences, whoop-de-doo, those thighs start to shrink. The hormones associated with lactation seem to be the *only* mechanism that activates the release of fat from the thighs.

By lowering their total body fat and doing muscle-shaping leg exercises, women can have attractive legs. But most women will ALWAYS have more fat in their thighs. It's part of being female.

It's sort of a "good news–bad news" joke. The good news is that female-type fat distribution isn't very dangerous because it isn't mobile fat. The bad news is that once it's deposited, it seems to stay there forever.

For men the joke is reversed. The good news is they can lose their belly fat very easily, but the bad news is it's dangerous fat. The fat cells in abdominal fat have a high turnover rate; they fill quickly when you overeat, but they release fat easily too. During stress, the abdominal fat cells become more active. If the stress is exercise, the fat released can be burned in the muscles. But what if the stress is emotional? Fat leaves the abdomen and travels through the bloodstream, but no muscle cells need the calories. So the fat ends up clinging to artery walls. Men with abdominal fat carry a potentially lethal package in their bellies. Any kind of emotional stress releases fat, which showers the heart and arteries.

Jiggly Thighs

One of the most common complaints I hear from women is, "No matter how hard I try, I can't get rid of my jiggly thighs." At 22 percent fat (considered a healthy level for women), most women still have some fat in their thighs. It jiggles because it builds up right under the skin surface. Abdominal fat, on the other hand, initially accumulates beneath the abdominal muscles. A man's stomach may be fat, but it is hard because the abdominal muscles are stretched taut over the fat. A woman's thighs may not be any fatter than a man's midsection, but they seem fatter because they're softer and jiggle more easily. Thighs usually slim down when total fat gets to 18 percent, but I've seen women with 15 percent fat (extraordinarily low for a female) whose bodies look too thin — yet their thighs still jiggle.

The Waist-to-Hip-Ratio Test

Belly fat is dangerous whether its owner is male or female. The potbellied man is at much greater risk of heart disease than a man who carries his fat all over his body. Male-type fat distribution, even if it occurs in a female, has been linked with cardiovascular disease, hypertension, high cholesterol and triglycerides, noninsulin-dependent diabetes, and even, in women, endometrial and ovarian cancers.

At what point does belly fat become dangerous? There is a simple home test you can do to assess your risk. It's called the waist-to-hip ratio. Despite its simplicity, the measurement is quite useful.

With a tape measure, measure your waist at its largest diameter above the belly button (on your skin without clothing). No fair cheating by sucking in! You may have to ask your spouse, "Where did my waist used to be?" Then measure your hips at their widest point. Then divide the waist measurement by the hip measurement. Ideally, if your hips are wider than your waist, the ratio is not more than 1.0. Since women naturally have broader hips than men, we expect their ratio to be a little lower. Men should be 0.9 or less. When they approach 1.0, they are just starting to develop a potbelly.

A man with a 34-inch waist and 38-inch hips would have a ratio of 0.9. If he gains weight, it would be quite typical for him to first distribute fat on both waist and hips. For example, he might add two inches to each measurement, for a 36-inch waist and 40-inch hips. Divide these two and it's still a 0.9. He can breathe a sigh of relief and say, "I'm not potbellied; I'm fat all over." If, however, he adds four inches of fat to his waist during the next few years, he gets 40 divided by 40, which equals 1.0. He has the beginnings of a potbelly and the increasing health hazards that go with it.

> **Belly fat is dangerous whether its owner is male or female.**

For a woman, a ratio of 0.8 or less is desirable. As with men, both measurements can increase equally, maintaining the same ratio. But when her waist measurement alone increases so that she approaches the male figures (pun intended) of 0.9, she's starting to get in trouble. Women who have repeatedly lost weight rapidly only to gain it all back usually regain in the belly until they have a ratio of 1.0 or more. Their bodies look more male, and they take on the male risk of cardiovascular problems.

The conclusion seems to be, when it comes to heart disease or hypertension, it's better to have a pear-shaped body than an apple-shaped body. Women with typical female fat distribution may hate the way it looks, but it doesn't seem to be a very dangerous kind of fat. It's potbelly fat we have to be afraid of.

Are Home Tests Really Useful?

Years ago, patients with high blood pressure were urged to visit their doctors frequently for blood pressure monitoring. Some went as often as once a month. The doctors and nurses assumed that only they could measure blood pressure accurately. And they had good reason to think so! The complexities of systolic and diastolic pressure, measured in millimeters of mercury, make that simple-looking test quite sophisticated.

Nonetheless, inexpensive kits for monitoring blood pressure at home were developed and marketed. Guess what happened? Home measurement produced better results. I don't mean that patients read or understood the machines better, but they measured themselves much more often and thus could tell their doctor what times of day and what conditions drove their blood pressure up. Patients could take the time to monitor themselves much more closely than the doctors could possibly do. Not only that, they took more interest in their condition, focusing more on how to control it. Testing their blood pressure themselves motivated them and helped them feel they were taking charge of their own health. Physicians, seeing the value in this, now encourage the use of home blood pressure machines. They know that measuring blood pressure just once in the doctor's office isn't very useful anyway. Blood pressure can be inaccurately high merely because you're in a strange place.

The point I'm making is that tests originally scorned by the experts can suddenly become quite respectable just by their volume of use. Your doctor's blood pressure machine may have cost two hundred dollars; you can buy one at the pharmacy for twenty-five dollars. Used regularly, yours may be more valuable in the long run by giving you and your doctor a day-by-day picture of your blood pressure.

> **Smart exercisers keep themselves motivated by using my three home fat and fitness tests.**

A similar evolution took place in the dietetic world. Dietitians used to feel that untrained individuals couldn't possibly analyze their own diet accurately. Again, they had good reason to believe so because of the intricacies of serving size, vitamin and mineral content, fiber content, and so on. But people began to use home methods of diet analysis found in books, including my own book *The Fit-or-Fat Target Diet*. Whammo! It happened again; a less accurate method gave more accurate results because it was used more often. And, even better, patients who analyzed their own diet habits became much more careful about what they ate.

I believe a similar change is in the making regarding the home tests described in this section. These tests don't involve computers with impressive printouts or machines with blinking lights, but you should not underrate their value. The waist-to-hip-ratio test, requiring only a tape measure, can tell you a lot. Just the process of finding your own pace will be fun for you, and once you have it figured out, you will feel more motivated to improve than you would with any expensive laboratory test. The same thing is happening with the skin calipers test. Even if it isn't as accurate as the water tank test, your ability to monitor yourself in the morning versus evening, summer versus Christmastime, will be far more powerful than some fancy computer printout.

The home tests in this section aren't meant to satisfy the technicians — they are for you. Remember the proverb: if you give a man a fish, you feed him for a day; if you teach him how to fish, you feed him for a lifetime.

9

Diet Tricks
for Performance

*Of all the dietary manipulations that have been
foisted on athletes, only the ones listed below
are worthy of discussion. Let the energy bars,
vitamin supplements, amino acids,
and pep pills remain with the hucksters
who started promoting them.*

How Carbohydrate Loading Works

The Carbo-Loading Regimen

The Effects of Caffeine

The Gut and Gas

How Carbohydrate Loading Works

Trained muscles have the ability to store more glycogen than untrained muscles. They also use less glycogen during exercise. Elite athletes, therefore, have a decided advantage over the rest of us. Since it's lack of glycogen that leads to muscle fatigue, they endure long, hard exercise better than we do. Moreover, by manipulating diet and exercise, they can pack even more glycogen into their muscles.

If I take off on a two-hour run, I want my muscles to burn fat efficiently because that is the primary fuel, but I don't want to run out of that glycogen kindling either. One way to do that is to have more glycogen in the muscles in the first place, a characteristic of elite athletes.

You can almost double the amount of glycogen that's typically found in skeletal muscles if you combine the right exercise with the proper dietary manipulation. We've all heard about the carbohydrate loading that marathon runners do before races. The technique was discovered in Finland by researchers working with cross-country skiers. They found that the skiers could endure much better and much longer and thus win races if they carbo-loaded. Basically, the concept is to do extreme exercise during the week prior to the marathon in order to deplete the muscles of glycogen. At the same time, the diet is very low in carbohydrate so that the glycogen isn't replenished. Two or three days prior to the race the athlete switches to a high-car-

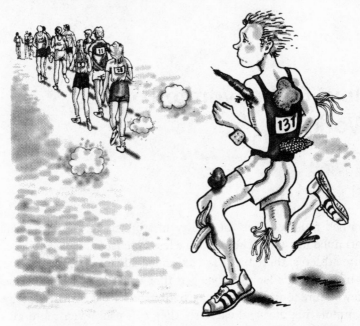

Gary tries new carbohydrate loading diet.

bohydrate diet. His starving muscles eagerly grab all the glucose they can get, producing above-normal amounts of glycogen.

There are problems with this technique, however. Let's say you like to run an occasional marathon, and you have a friend who is an elite marathon runner. Your friend might carbo-load before his next marathon and do very, very well. You decide to try it before your next marathon, and you do very, very poorly. Your muscles are not in the extremely hypersensitive state that allows them to absorb glucose quickly and convert it into glycogen efficiently. Instead it goes right to the fat cells, which will always accept glucose molecules and convert them into fat molecules. For the average athlete carbohydrate loading often backfires; instead of running faster, he runs slower. When that happens, the person makes the mistake of claiming that the technique doesn't work at all. It *does* work — if you are fit enough.

There are other problems. Any time you put glycogen in a muscle cell, it demands a little bit of water. For every molecule of glycogen stored, three molecules of water are needed. Sometimes even elite athletes run less well after carbohydrate loading because the extra water increases their weight and has a stiffening effect on the muscles. So! Even if you can store more glycogen, the trick may still backfire because of the increased water storage.

> **You can almost double the amount of glycogen in muscle by manipulating exercise and diet.**

Despite these drawbacks, carbo-loading does work for elite athletes. Of all the dietary tricks — vitamin pills, pep pills, amino acids, and so on — that are advised, pushed, and marketed to athletes, the only one that's ever been shown to have scientific credibility is carbohydrate loading. It does work, but only if you're very fit. And even the very fit have to experiment with it, because everyone responds to carbohydrates a little differently. It may turn out that carbohydrate loading just doesn't work for you. If several attempts result in lower performance, you must accept the fact that you aren't a glycogen storer.

If you decide that carbo-loading is for you, and you're willing to put up with all the possible problems associated with it, please keep in mind that this manipulation improves endurance, not speed. Intensity can be improved only through training. Also remember that "hitting the wall," the sudden fatigue we believe is caused by running out of glycogen, only occurs in long-distance events that last two hours or more. It's foolish to carbo-load for a six-mile race.

The Carbo-Loading Regimen

The classic form of carbohydrate loading (dietary stripping followed by supercompensation) was popular in the 1960s and '70s, but athletes were warned not to try it more than a couple times a year because it often caused dizziness, lack of energy, and hallucinations. The most likely reason for these symptoms is depletion of carbohydrate in the brain (which must have glucose for energy) and the conversion of body protein into glucose.

New research in the late 1970s showed that carbo-loading did not have to be so strict. The preliminary stripping of carbohydrates from the diet is unnecessary. Instead of cutting way back to 10 percent carbohydrate, you can eat a normal 50–60 percent carbohydrate diet, then pump it up to 70 percent about six days before a race. The muscles will overload on glycogen just as if they had been depleted. People on a 50 percent carbohydrate diet will raise their glycogen levels just as much as those who cut back to 10 percent. This change eliminates the harmful side effects mentioned earlier and results in better long-term performance. Additionally, tapering off gradually on exercise has been shown to be more effective than engaging in bouts of exhaustive exercise followed by periods of rest. These two things — exercise tapering coupled with a 50 percent carbohydrate diet that is gradually increased to 70 percent — will raise glycogen levels far above normal levels.

Today the commonly recommended tapering/carbohydrate-loading program is as shown in the table.

Days before race	Exercise session	Intensity	Diet — percentage of carbohydrate
6–7	90 min.	Hard	50–60%
5	40–60 min.	Moderate	50–60%
4	30–40 min.	Moderate	60–70%
3	20–30 min.	Moderate	70%
2	20 min.	Mild	70%
1	Rest		70%
Race day	Stretch and warm up		Pre-race meal of 500–800 calories of carbohydrate

Eager first-time loaders sometimes ask if eating more than 70 percent carbohydrate will increase their glycogen storage even more. Trust me, it won't. Those of you who have tried a 70 percent carbohydrate diet are probably chuckling at the thought of eating even more. It's HARD to eat that much carbohydrate, isn't it? If you ate more, you'd never get away from the table. If you aren't used to high-fiber eating, don't try it just before a race. You are too likely to suffer some gastric distress.

High-fiber eating takes a lot of time because you have to eat an enormous amount of sheer bulk. Plan on eating several times a day — you just can't do it in three sittings. Carbohydrate loading means grazing on grains, cereals, fruits, and vegetables — ALL DAY LONG. Too often, athletes cheat themselves out of necessary calories because they just get tired of chewing! A typical male needs approximately 2,700 calories a day. If he's training hard for a marathon, he needs about 2,000 more calories to meet the additional energy requirements. A quart of ice cream would supply an extra 2,000 calories but would defeat the purpose because those are concentrated fat calories. Let's take a look at a typical day of carbo-loading:

High-Carbohydrate (70%) Menu

	Serving size	Carbohydrate (grams)	Calories
Breakfast			
Corn flakes	2 cups	48	220
Nonfat milk	2 cups	24	180
Banana	1 large	30	115
Whole-wheat toast	3 slices	42	195
Jelly	3 tsp.	30	120
Orange juice	2 cups	50	226
Snack (immediately after workout)			
After-exercise carbohydrate beverage	1 cup	50	200
Snack (1 hour after workout)			
Pear	2 medium	50	200
Lunch			
Two sandwiches made of:			
whole-wheat bread	4 slices	56	260
sliced turkey breast	7.2 oz.	0	200
tomato, sliced	1 medium	6	26
shredded lettuce	½ cup	2	5
low-fat American cheese	4 oz.	4	200
Carrot and celery sticks	1 carrot, 1 stalk celery	9	35
Apple juice	2 cups	58	240
Almond granola bar	1	15	110
Snack			
Low-fat fruit-flavored yogurt	1 cup	42	230
Bagel	1	30	165

	Serving size	Carbohydrate (grams)	Calories
Dinner			
Spaghetti with meatless sauce	3 cups cooked	111	780
Mixed green salad (lettuce, tomatoes, broccoli, mushrooms, green onions, carrots)	2 cups	17	80
Salad dressing, low-calorie	4 tbsp.	4	40
Roll	2 medium	42	240
Margarine	2 tbsp.	0	200
Green beans	2 cups	16	80
Cantaloupe	½	20	80
Nonfat skim milk	2 cups	24	180
Snack			
Popcorn, no oil	3 cups	15	75
Apple juice	1 cup	29	120
		790	4,667

Total calories 4,667

Total carbohydrate calories 3,160*

Percentage of carbohydrate calories 68%**

---

*To calculate carbohydrate calories, multiply grams of carbohydrate by 4
(790 × 4 = 3,160)
**To calculate percentage of carbohydrate calories, divide carbohydrate calories by total calories
(3,160 ÷ 4,667 = .677 or, rounded off, 68%)

As you can see, this is a tremendous quantity of food; the menu should give you a better understanding of how hard it is to get 70 percent of your calories from carbohydrates. Since there's no additional payoff in terms of increased glycogen storage, eating more than 70 percent just isn't practical.

The Effects of Caffeine

Caffeine stimulates the release of fatty acids into the blood. With more fatty acids available, the muscles need less glucose. A few years ago it was popular for marathon runners to take caffeine before a marathon, hoping that the extra fatty acids would be used as fuel, thus saving their limited glycogen supply. The caffeine did seem to help at first, but it exacerbated other long-distance running problems. One drawback is that caffeine is a diuretic and thus promotes water loss from the body; taking caffeine on a hot day increases the risk of dehydration and heat exhaustion.

Another problem with caffeine for endurance events is that it competes with insulin. Many runners go on high-carbohydrate diets and eat sugary foods or drinks in order to maintain muscle glycogen. The resultant high blood sugar keeps blood insulin levels high, which inhibits the release of fatty acids from fat cells. Caffeine stimulates the release of fatty acids, while insulin does the opposite. Runners are faced with a Catch-22. Should they drink coffee to raise their fatty acid levels or eat lots of carbohydrate to increase glycogen levels? For a few years there was lots of personal experimentation.

Unfortunately, caffeine contributes to tension and nervousness before a race, and it also irritates the bowel. If you add pre-race nerves to caffeine nerves to bowel irritation, you get diarrhea. Runners found that having to step behind a tree in the middle of a race decreased their speed a lot more than the extra fatty acids increased their speed.

Since caffeine promotes the release of fatty acids, why not use it for weight loss? I can just picture the next weight-loss rip-off scheme: "Jive up your weight loss with java." Here's the catch: if fatty acids are released from fat pads but not *used* by muscle, they go right back to other fat pads. Like some poor soul all dressed up for the party with nowhere to go, the fatty acids flit from muscle to muscle, saying, "How about we get together and make some action?" To which the lazy muscle replies, "Buzz off, kid. We don't exercise. We just drink coffee." Pretty soon, the fatty acids get tired of being rejected and scoot on back to the fat pads to be with all their friends. A release of fatty acids doesn't result in weight loss unless the fatty acids are burned up.

What about other effects of caffeine? A few years back newspapers were filled with articles on the hazards of caffeine to unborn babies. And they were true! Your baby *will* have missing toes if you drink eighty-seven cups of coffee a day. Ridiculous, isn't it? The data was based on rat studies in which the rats were force-fed the equivalent of eighty-seven cups of coffee a day.

Coffee or caffeine consumption has also been linked with cancer. In 1981 the Harvard School of Public Health suggested that more than half of the 20,000 cases of pancreatic cancer occurring in the United States every year might be linked to coffee drinking. Even people drinking as few as one or two cups a day were at risk. Five years later *the same research group* reversed their findings, stating that they could find no connection between caffeine or coffee consumption and pancreatic cancer. Breast cancer and bladder cancer have likewise been shown to have no connection with caffeine consumption.

Other early research scared the public with claims that caffeine increased the risk of heart disease, raised cholesterol levels, or caused fibrocystic breast disease. But again, subsequent studies could not validate the earlier claims. In fact, if you were to wade through all the research on caffeine you'd go crazy. There are studies that show a link between coffee drinking and cholesterol in men aged forty to forty-five (but not thirty-five to forty or forty-five to fifty) who drink four cups of coffee a day (but not three cups or five cups). There are fat-people studies, male-female studies, probably even aborigine studies. I'm sure there are even data on coffee-drinking five-year-old three-toed sloths, but I haven't come across it yet, thank God.

Surprisingly, caffeine seems to have a positive effect on people who suffer from bronchial asthma. Long-term moderate consumption of coffee (one or two cups a day) not only eases their symptoms, it may actually prevent their recurrence. In a survey of 70,000 adults, those who drank up to three cups of coffee a day experienced 27 percent fewer asthma attacks than those who did not drink coffee. This research has to be taken with a grain of salt; other lifestyle factors in the population surveyed may have influenced the results.

If coffee and tea were discovered today, the FDA would never release them to the market!

Most research currently agrees that a breast-feeding woman should limit her caffeine intake. Caffeine makes its way into breast milk, to which the nursing infant responds with a higher respiratory rate and increased urine output. Most mothers don't enjoy panting, peeing, irritable babies. And it takes from *two to twelve days* for the little bugger to process the caffeine out of his system!

After all this talk about caffeine studies and refuted caffeine studies, it's hard to make a definitive statement. The heavy coffee drinker says, "Nothing's been proven, so leave me alone." Obviously that is not true. Caffeine is a very powerful drug with quick and provable effects on the central nervous system, the peripheral nervous system, and the gut. It is used in many prescription and over-the-counter pills. It is also a habituating drug; you have to take more and more to get the same effects. If coffee and tea were discovered today, the FDA would never release them to the market. Personally, I treat coffee the way I treat alcohol. A little bit now and then MAY be okay. But overdo and you are asking for trouble.

How Much Caffeine Does It Have?

Substance	Milligrams of caffeine
Coffee	
drip, 8 oz.	150–180
perked, 8 oz.	125
instant, 8 oz.	30–120
decaffeinated, 8 oz.	2–8
Tea	
brewed, 8 oz.	20–100
instant, 8 oz.	30–70
Soft drinks	
Mountain Dew, 12 oz.	54
colas, 12 oz.	36–46
Other	
hot cocoa, 8 oz.	4–8
semisweet chocolate, 1 oz.	14
Vivarin, 1 tablet	200
No-Doz, 1 tablet	100
Excedrin, 1 tablet	75
Anacin, 1 tablet	32
Midol, 1 tablet	32

The Gut and Gas

This chapter isn't about a true dietary manipulation, but if you're trying some carbo-loading or caffeine tricks with your diet, you might find it fun to read.

High-fiber diets tend to produce a lot of intestinal gas, which sometimes can be so uncomfortable that it inhibits you from exercising. We seem to be between a rock and hard place. All competent nutrition experts urge us to eat less fat and more complex carbohydrates such as vegetables, whole-grain breads, and cereals. But complex carbohydrates are only partially digestible, and as a result gas is produced in the bowel, especially the large intestine.

Everybody on a high-fiber diet produces gas, but in some people it doesn't have a bad odor and is passed without conse-'quence. It isn't the production of gas that causes the problems, it's the entrapment of gas when the normal passage is restricted.

The large intestine is only five feet long, but it has some very sharp bends, or flexures. One of these is on the right side of the abdomen beneath the liver. Another is beneath the stomach on the left side. Tiny muscles embedded in the wall of the intestine help squeeze food along. These muscles are activated by nerves. When you get a case of "nerves" from drinking coffee, smoking, or tension, the natural flexure in the large intestine is twisted further and sometimes the passage is shut off altogether. Those of us who are not routine coffee drinkers find that an occasional cup makes our stomachs jumpy. It hyperirritates the bowel, and the result is that normal gas production, which didn't cause a problem yesterday, causes a problem today.

> **If you get gas from some foods,
> the problem may not be the food.**

I'm not saying that gas in the gut can be stopped. If you're eating a high-fiber diet, you're going to produce gas, but the gas may not bother you unless something else irritates the bowel to the point of trapping the gas. Don't give up high-fiber food because of the distension that comes with it. It may very well be something else that is irritating your bowel, like coffee, cigarettes, or even stress.

This whole discussion adds yet another dimension to my prejudice about exercise. You may be thinking, "Oh-oh, if he tells me fit people have less gas than fat people, I'm closing this book right now!" I won't go that far, but fit people DO have less stress in their lives and better control of their stress when it does occur. They DO tend to be less compulsive. They DO tend to avoid coffee and alcohol and cigarettes. They're calm about their environment, their habits, and themselves.

10

Sweating and Dehydration

The Physiology of Sweating

The sole purpose of sweating is to cool the body. When your body temperature rises because of exercise, fever, or the heat of the day, your heart responds by pumping faster to move blood around to all the organs more quickly and absorb their heat. If it's really hot or you're exercising strenuously, the blood itself gets too warm to cool off hot organs, and at that point your "built-in shower," the sweating reflex, kicks in.

Now picture the following. Dry your hand thoroughly, hold it out palm up, and place one drop of water in the middle. Picture four or five of us standing around, staring at the drop of water, waiting for it to disappear. Suddenly, like Houdini, poof! It's gone! This visible, tangible droplet of water has evaporated into thin air. It takes calories — heat energy — to make this miracle happen, *lots* of heat energy. Picture your body covered with such droplets, disappearing one by one. The amount of heat one water droplet has to absorb in order to evaporate into the atmosphere is awesome; and for a thousand droplets to evaporate, it's turbo-awesome. When you exercise hard, you produce enough heat to evaporate two quarts of water in one hour. Imagine two quarts of water in a pan on your stove. Think of the heat required to boil it all until the pan is dry. You produce that much heat in one hour of hard exercise AND the sweating mechanism can make that much heat disappear in one hour — awesome. The point is that water evaporating from the skin has a fantastic cooling effect on the skin and therefore on the blood flowing near the skin.

While you're sitting reading this book, your body is churning away on all kinds of metabolic activities, like digesting dinner or repairing muscles from this morning's run. Whatever it's doing, it has to burn calories. The word "burn" is appropriate because heat is produced. Even when you're just sitting, you produce enough heat to raise your body temperature two or three degrees an hour! During exercise the body produces ten to fifteen times as much heat. If there were no mechanism for dissipating this heat, you'd be a fried egg in no time.

> **If you didn't sweat during exercise,
> you'd be a fried egg in minutes!**

To get rid of the extra heat produced by exercise, capillaries just under the skin open up, allowing the heat to get closer to the surface. That's why you're flushed and red after exercise.

Pretty soon the body has a new problem to deal with — dehydration. Most of the water lost by sweating is drawn from the blood. An average man has about eleven pints of blood, which is about eleven pounds. If he loses six pounds playing tennis in the sun, you can figure that at least half of that is water from the blood, dropping his blood volume 27 percent. Suppose you're playing tennis on a hot day, but you don't stop for a drink between sets. After a while you start missing easy shots. Your muscles don't respond quickly. What's happened is that the blood has become less watery and more sludgy. In this state it can't move as easily, it can't pick up oxygen easily when it goes through the lungs, and it doesn't give up the oxygen readily when it gets to the muscles. The muscles, deprived of oxygen, perform less well. Clumsiness, dizziness, and disorientation are fast approaching. In this state you tend to disregard your friend's warnings about your deteriorating condition.

If you continue to exercise in spite of being dehydrated, the muscles get frantic. "We've GOT to have oxygen in here! Don't slow down the blood supply!" To assure that blood gets to the muscles in your dehydrated state, the flow of blood to the skin decreases and sweating diminishes in order to conserve water. At the very time when body heat is building up dangerously and the sweating mechanism is most needed, sweating is prevented and body temperature can rise very quickly. Victims of heat stroke are hot to the touch, yet their skin is dry.

One way to gauge how much water you're losing is to weigh yourself after exercising. If you lose 4 percent of your weight during exercise, you've lost 18 to 20 percent of your body water. For every pound lost during exercise, replace with a pint — two cups — of water. (Easy to remember with the rhyme "A pint's a pound the world around.")

Here are the rules for replacing fluids lost during exercise:

1. Drink a cup of water about a half hour before exercising.
2. Drink 3 to 6 ounces of fluid every fifteen or twenty minutes during the exercise. (If the exercise only lasts twenty to thirty minutes this isn't necessary.)
3. Don't wait until you're thirsty. Follow a water replenishment schedule. If you wait until you notice your thirst, you're already becoming dehydrated.
4. Drink cool fluids. Fluids at 40 to 50 degrees F. pass through the stomach and into the bloodstream more quickly than warm or ice-cold beverages.
5. After exercise, fruit juices or sports drinks are better than water for rehydration.

To avoid heat exhaustion here are some other points to remember:

- Wear clothing that allows the body to breathe.
- Don't exercise when you have a fever.
- On very hot days, exercise in the early morning or late evening. Better yet, go swimming!

Who Sweats More —
Fit People or Fat People?

Fit people excel at resisting fluctuations in their core temperature. When they exercise mildly on a moderately hot day, they get rid of heat so efficiently that their core temperature doesn't change. Unfit people, in the same conditions, start to accumulate core heat fairly quickly, triggering the sweating mechanism. That's why fat, unfit people appear to sweat sooner and more copiously than fit people. We have all seen fat people sweating like crazy on a mildly hot day, which tends to make us think that it's the fat causing the sweating. In fact, low fitness is more the cause. Equally fit male and female athletes sweat the same even though females almost always have more fat.

You'd think that an out-of-shape person would sweat more than a fit person, yet actually it's just the opposite. That fact is not apparent because the fit person keeps his core temperature in check better. But if his core temperature starts to rise in spite of his superior system, the fit person starts sweating immediately. It's as if his sweat mechanism, like all his other bodily mechanisms, is more in tune with his needs. He resists any initial rise in core temperature, but if it does rise he compensates more quickly.

Suppose three groups of people are asked to run on a hot day. One group consists of trained, fit runners who regularly exercise in hot weather. The second group are also trained runners, but they've just flown in from Alaska and aren't used to the heat. And the third group are couch potatoes who happened to be on the same Alaskan flight with the runners. In other words, they're unfit *and* unused to the heat.

If we were to take the internal core temperature of all three groups during the run, we'd find that sweating kicks in at about 98.9 degrees in the fit, acclimated runners. In the fit Alaskan runners sweating starts at a slightly higher temperature, 99.5 degrees. And the couch potatoes don't start sweating until their internal temperature gets up to 99.9 degrees. The fitter and more acclimated the runner, the sooner the sweat response begins. Unfit people heat up faster than fit people, but their sweating mechanisms take longer to get started. In general, fit people are more efficient at cooling their bodies.

Ultra-Athletes Sweat Too Much!

Very fit athletes handle cold less well than one might expect. They not only lack the fat that acts as insulation in cold conditions, their core temperatures drop faster than those of nonathletes. They are so efficient at getting rid of heat that they lose heat when they shouldn't. As a result, ultra-athletes are more at risk in the cold.

Myths about Sweating

While jogging on a hot day, I passed a man who was all bundled up in plastic and towels. I couldn't resist asking him, "Say, uh, why are you dressed like that on such a hot day?" He replied, with a withering look, "To sweat off fat, of course."

Such people think that when they sweat they are losing lots of fat. Not true. They are losing water. How much fat you lose depends on how well your muscles are trained to burn the stuff, and that depends on how aerobically fit you are. You can't "sweat off" fat. Yes, that guy will lose *weight* by sweating — water weight. He'll become a dehydrated fat person.

People who put on lots of clothing and wrap towels around their necks when they exercise are defeating the purpose of sweating. They raise their body temperature but don't allow the sweat to evaporate and cool the body. It's okay to wear extra clothing during your warm-up, but you should shed the outer layers as your body temperature rises. You want a warmed-up body, not an overheated one. Let your body sweat and cool naturally. The idea that we must "work up a good sweat" by using saunas or wearing plastic jogging suits is just plain silly and potentially dangerous.

Another common belief is that sweating rids the body of toxins. Sweat is nothing more than water, salts, and urea. The body isn't detoxified when it sweats; the only thing it gets rid of is water and a few salts.

It was popular several years ago to take salt tablets. This turned out to be as effective as fixing a broken hinge with a

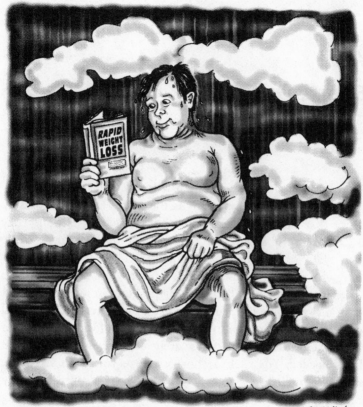

Fat boils at 360°!

sledgehammer. The salts lost during a thirty- to forty-five-minute session of moderate exercise are negligible. They are easily replaced in the first postexercise meal. If you exercise at high intensity for several hours, taking a sports drink or electrolyte drink during and after the activity can be helpful (see "Sports Drinks").

The bottom line is: don't worry about how much you sweat. Some people sweat more than others, just as some people drool more when they go to the dentist. Just drink lots of fluid and avoid overheating.

Sports Drinks

Sports drinks are the "in" thing with the sweat generation — they're becoming as important as the proper shoes. There is no doubt that they are effective in combating dehydration. They are also a useful sugar source during endurance events. While their claims of replacing electrolytes and providing a "super energy" supply are dubious, they are very effective at getting water into the body, which is a big problem in long events.

For a twenty- to thirty-minute exercise, water works as well to avoid dehydration as anything else. A cup of water a half hour before exercise and a cup immediately after exercise should be all that's needed. For such a short exercise you don't need the calories provided in a sports drink, nor do you need to worry about replacing minerals. The little sodium you lose during twenty to thirty minutes of moderate exercise is easily replaced with a normal diet.

Sports drinks are designed for longer, harder events. Studies have shown that after long bouts of exercise or hard work, sports drinks rehydrate you faster and more thoroughly than water alone. Drinking water tends to shut down the thirst mechanism, so most people stop drinking when they are only 68 percent rehydrated. Water also stimulates the production of urine, something you *do not* want more of when you are dehydrated. The minerals in sports drinks, particularly sodium, prolong your thirst, so you are more likely to keep drinking until fully rehydrated. The minerals also inhibit urine production. People who rehydrate with a sodium solution keep drinking until they're about 82 percent rehydrated.

Drinking a sports drink containing glucose and other sugars *before* an event presents a problem. The sugar causes blood insulin to rise, and insulin inhibits the release of fatty acids from fat cells. For the first half hour of the event, your fat cells won't release the primary fuel. With fatty acids unavailable, your muscles are forced to use stored glycogen and then the sugar in the blood. This means that sugar supplies are burned up even more quickly than normal. Taking a sugar drink so you won't run out of sugar will, in fact, cause you to run out of sugar sooner! This won't happen if you take the drink during or after exercise because the fatty acids have already entered the bloodstream.

> **"When is the best time for a sports drink — before, during, or after exercise?"**

The sugar in a sports drink consumed during exercise is easily tolerated and, in fact, enhances performance by prolonging endurance. Drinking a sports drink every fifteen to twenty minutes during exercise provides a steady trickle of glucose that spares the glycogen in the muscle.

The trick is to find a drink that has enough glucose to be useful to the muscles but not so much that it can't be absorbed quickly. Sports drinks containing 5 to 7 percent glucose apparently have just that effect. Fruit juices usually contain 10 percent or more glucose and fructose, making it more difficult to absorb them.

When sugars aren't absorbed rapidly, gastric distress and diarrhea can result. Most of us know that salt attracts water. In a humid environment, the salt in a shaker gets all caked together. Sugar has similar properties. So, when a sugary drink gets to the intestinal tract, it draws water out of the bloodstream into the intestine. Sports drinks with glucose are absorbed into the bloodstream before this intestinal flooding can occur. Sugar drinks containing fructose (fruit juices) remain in the gut longer and draw in substantial amounts of water, which can lead to cramping and diarrhea.

Why Is Glucose Absorbed Faster than Fructose?

Glucose and fructose molecules are exactly the same size. They each contain six atoms of carbon, twelve atoms of hydrogen, and six atoms of oxygen. The only difference between them is the way the carbon, hydrogen, and oxygen are hooked to each other. You'd think that because they're the same size, they would be absorbed at the same rate. Not so. Glucose molecules enter the bloodstream much faster than fructose.

When any substance enters the small intestine it needs a way to get into the bloodstream. The intestinal wall has a "glucose pump" that actively sucks up glucose and spits it out into the bloodstream. Glucose also drags along a lot of water with it when it's transported through the intestinal wall. In fact, it's been shown that water coupled with glucose enters the bloodstream faster than water alone. This is one of the reasons sports drinks rehydrate you quicker than water.

Fructose, on the other hand, has to wait in line like everything else, more or less leaking through the intestinal wall into the bloodstream. Then, like some weary traveler after a long flight, it needs to go through customs — the liver. There it is delayed for several minutes while some of its molecules are switched around so it can be converted into glucose.

To avoid flooding, some sports drinks are made with glucose polymers — glucose molecules strung together into one larger molecule. Proponents of glucose polymers argue that they tend to moderate fluctuations in blood sugar and do not flood the intestine. But studies so far indicate that they have no advantage in metabolic action or water balance. Glucose and glucose polymers appear to be equal in their ability to enhance performance and rehydrate the body.

What about the other ingredients in sports drinks? All the ads for these drinks brag about their electrolytes. What are they? Do we need them?

Electrolytes are simply minerals. When minerals dissolve in the bloodstream, they form salts that take on an electrical charge. In a sense, they're like little batteries. Without these batteries, nerve impulses could not be conducted; the brain couldn't make all its phone calls directing body movement and function. Electrolytes are also responsible for maintaining fluid levels in the body by regulating the water balance inside and outside cells. Even the body's delicate acid/alkaline balance is carefully monitored and controlled in part by electrolytes.

Any mineral can be an electrolyte, but the main ones are sodium, potassium, and chloride. If you look on a sports drink label, you'll see that these are the usual "electrolytes" added, although some drinks also contain calcium, magnesium, and phosphorus. By calling them electrolytes, manufacturers make a lot more money from the naive consumer than if the label just said "minerals added."

When you consider how essential electrolytes are to survival, it's scary to think that you could sweat them away during exercise. But the truth is, unless you're doing an ultra-endurance event like a fifty-mile run or a one-hundred-mile bicycle race, you don't lose very many electrolytes.

You probably don't need the electrolytes in sports drinks, but I doubt that they do any harm, for the amounts added are minuscule. One glass of most sports beverages contains the same amount of sodium as a glass of milk and the same amount of potassium as one bite of a banana. During very heavy, strenuous work or exercise in which you lose enormous quantities of sweat, then *perhaps* your electrolytes need to be replenished. But as you remember from our earlier discussion, it's the replacement of water that is critical. As far as I can tell, the true value of electrolyte drinks is that they tend to keep you thirsty and enhance flavor so you drink more.

Now, which sports drink is best? There are several on the market, and new ones come out all the time. You might have to experiment with several brands and flavors to find one you like. Remember, the key issue here is rehydration. The better it tastes, the more you're going to drink.

You also need to think about the concentration of the drink. A solution of 5–7 percent glucose has been the standard for endurance events lasting one to three hours. New on the market are sports drinks with 1–3 percent glucose. These are geared toward the recreational athlete who engages in moderate, shorter exercise sessions. As I said before, water will rehydrate you just fine under these circumstances, but some people prefer the flavored beverage and will drink more of it.

Also new are superconcentrated solutions of 15–25 percent glucose for the "Ironman"-type athletes, those who run hundred-mile races or bicycle for days at a time or compete in grueling, all-day triathlons. Laboratory experiments indicate that these beverages provide the energy so essential for such events; however, they create gastric problems for many people, making them difficult to tolerate. In any case, don't use these beverages until well into the race, probably after one hour of hard work.

11

How to Make More Muscle

You don't have to be a bodybuilder to want more muscle. Muscle does so much for you, it pays to have a lot of it.

How Much Protein Do We Really Need?

Do Weightlifters Need Extra Protein?

The Amino Acid Pool

How Do Muscles Grow?

Fast Twitch, Slow Twitch

More about Lactic Acid

Do Men Have More Fast-Twitch Fibers?

Does the Type of Training Determine Fiber Type?

Can You Switch Your Twitch?

The Fat Weightlifter

Anabolic Steroids

How Much Protein Do We Really Need?

The human body needs about 25–30 grams of protein every day to keep hair, skin, and tissues in good repair. The reason for the range is mostly size. Smaller people need 25 grams a day, and larger people, typically men, need a bit more, up to 30 grams per day. The research to prove this has been done many times in laboratories all over the world. The conclusions are not based on research from one particular laboratory or one particular group of people but have been gathered from research repeated over and over.

Why, then, is the Recommended Daily Allowance for protein 50 to 60 grams per day? It's because the RDA is doubled in case someone, somewhere, needs extra protein either because his body is different or because he has weird food habits. For example, consider a starving graduate student living on peanut butter. Peanut butter contains lots of protein, but it's not a "perfect" protein, so the body doesn't use it perfectly or completely. What if a woman eats 25 grams of perfect protein, but she is a weightlifter? And has a broken leg? And is pregnant? All of these add to her daily requirement for protein, but the RDA of 50 grams more than covers the increase.

So the RDA for protein, as for most of the vitamins and minerals, is doubled to cover worst-case scenarios. For 99.9 percent of the population, 25 to 30 grams of protein is more than adequate to build and repair all the tissues and keep us as

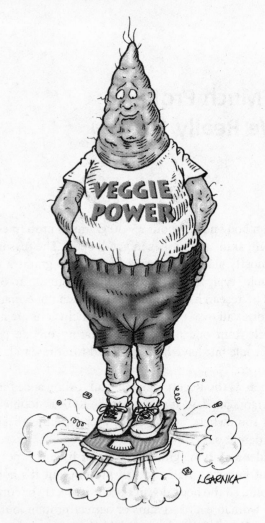

**Fred suspects he may have to do
more than just cut out meat......**

healthy as can be. It's only for that one tenth of one percent of
the population that we have the doubled RDA.

   Protein isn't hard to get. Most people eat far more than the body needs. A small hamburger from a fast-food place has about 23 grams of protein just in the meat alone. A slice of cheese adds another 7 grams, and a good whole-wheat bun another 2.5 grams. There's over 30 grams of protein in that one lousy cheeseburger. An ordinary can of tuna fish contains 50 grams of protein — double what you need for a day.

All meats are high in protein. A small serving of liver (about the size of a McDonald's hamburger) has 25 grams of protein. A similar serving of sirloin steak also has 25 grams. The same quantity of lean ham provides 28 grams. A glass of milk has 8 grams of protein, an egg has 6, and whole-wheat toast has 2, so a breakfast of a couple of eggs, two slices of toast, and a glass of milk provides almost the whole protein requirement for a day.

Do vegetarians get enough protein?

There's no doubt that animal protein sticks to the human body better than protein from other sources. If it looks like me, it probably will stick to me. I may not look like a goat, but I look more like a goat than like a carrot or a slice of bread. The highest-quality protein of all is egg protein. After all, when you eat an egg you're getting beak protein, feather protein — the whole bird! The problem with animal products is the fat. It's a two-edged sword. Animal products have the best and the most protein but also the highest fat content. And animal fat sticks to me just as well as animal protein does. The fat in meats and cheeses is much more likely to stick to your body than oils taken from vegetables and grains.

While it's easy to get enough protein from animal products, vegetarians have to try a little harder. Animal products contain complete proteins, meaning that all the amino acids needed for any protein construction job are available. If you're a vegetarian, your liver needs to do a little more mixing and matching to come up with proteins your body can use. After protein is digested, its amino acid components are stored in various "amino acid pools" in the liver, blood, and muscles. The amino acids in these pools can be connected to form whatever type of protein the body happens to need at a particular time.

If you eat mashed potatoes, a poor source of protein, the liver rummages around until it comes up with some suitable amino acids that can be hooked to the amino acids of the mashed potatoes to become a high-quality muscle-building protein. Rice and beans contain two different kinds of incomplete protein. If you eat just rice or just beans, the liver can't do much with the amino acids, but in combination their proteins make up a complete protein. This was not understood for a long time. People said, "Oh! I must have animal protein every day." But we now know that's not necessary. Mixing two or three incomplete proteins, like whole-wheat bread with peanut butter, makes it unnecessary to have animal protein at all.

Some people still don't believe we get enough protein, so let's look at how the researchers came up with the RDA's. When I was in graduate school, I was a guinea pig in some of the RDA studies. I was used just like a rat to make sure that the studies done on rats were comparable to those done on humans. If you were to participate in one of those studies as either a guinea pig or a researcher, you'd have a lot more respect for the Recommended Daily Allowances. The studies teach a great deal about how proteins are used, where they go, and why one protein is better than another. The RDA's are not printed by government agencies as a con job. They represent the combined wisdom of the very best nutritionists throughout the world.

The amount of protein the body uses is determined through nitrogen-balance studies, which are tedious and not much fun. Since protein, unlike fat and carbohydrate, contains nitrogen, the amount of protein the body uses each day can be ascertained by measuring how much nitrogen is eaten and how much is excreted. The nitrogen content of every morsel of food consumed as well as of everything that comes out — not only in urine but also in feces, sweat, menses, semen, and even hair and whiskers — must be carefully measured. Normally people are in nitrogen balance; that is, the amount that goes in each day equals the amount that comes out. Growing children and weight-lifters are often in positive nitrogen balance, which means that the body is retaining more protein than it is excreting. People with disease or under stress go into negative nitrogen balance.

The nitrogen studies measure exactly how much protein a person needs to stay in nitrogen balance. Obviously, a growing child needs a lot more protein than someone who is not growing. Someone repairing a broken leg also requires more.

The studies concluded that the amount of protein the body needs is not subject to debate. The RDA for protein is a very sensible number. It accounts for the extra you need if you're eating incomplete protein or lifting weights or repairing a broken leg or making a baby.

Do Weightlifters Need Extra Protein?

Pregnant women need far more protein than weightlifters. So do people with broken legs and long-distance runners. Bodybuilders and weightlifters DO need more protein, but not that much more.

The maximum muscle mass the human body can add in one week is one pound. That is the upper limit of the muscle fibers' capacity to make protein into muscle; any protein beyond that is simply converted to fat. Muscle on the body is exactly like the sirloin steaks you buy at the grocery store. If you took a pound of sirloin steak to a chemist to analyze, he'd find that it contained just over 100 grams of protein. A bodybuilder who wants to add a pound of extra muscle to his body needs 100 grams of protein. He could do that in a week by consuming 15 extra grams of protein per day. One cup of nonfat yogurt has 13 grams of protein, so you can see it isn't too difficult to meet the additional requirements.

Interestingly, endurance athletes need more protein than bodybuilders because apparently they use amino acids as fuel. We used to think that only fat and glucose were used for energy, but it's been shown that 5 to 10 percent of the energy needs of long-distance runners are supplied by amino acids. If they're exercising more than sixty minutes a day, their protein requirement may increase by as much as 67 percent.

Weightlifters and bodybuilders need only about 12 percent

more protein than people who don't exercise. Weightlifters don't "burn" protein like endurance athletes; they use it more sparingly to synthesize new muscle tissue.

If weightlifters and bodybuilders can build only a pound of muscle a week, why do some seem to gain much more than that on high-protein diets? They eat dozens of eggs, drink gallons of milk, and tear into steaks and cheeses, and many of them DO build more muscle than expected. Are the researchers wrong? Does the protein in all those foods build more muscle than expected?

> **Weightlifters need less protein than marathoners.**

The party-line nutrition advice on this point has consistently been that you can't utilize more than so much protein, so eating all those animal products isn't going to enhance your muscles. The party line is wrong! Animal products contain fats, and animal fats have steroids that enhance muscle growth.

We'll look at the relationship between steroids and muscle growth later on; the point here is that eating lots of meats, cheese, and eggs does make muscles grow bigger. But it's not the protein in these foods that stimulates muscle growth — it's the steroids in the fat. When ranchers want to "beef up" their cattle, they put the steroid DES, diethylstilbestrol, in cattle feed. Steroids, whether natural in animal products or synthesized for black-market drugs, make muscles absorb more protein than normal ("beefing" them up) but also add more fat. When weightlifters beef up they think they are only adding protein to their muscles, but ranchers know that beefing up adds protein and fat — that's what well-marbled steaks are.

The Amino Acid Pool

There is a special group of men who paint the Golden Gate Bridge in San Francisco. They start at one end of the bridge and slowly scrape and paint their way across. It takes a long time because there is a lot of steel and a lot of rust from the salty air. By the time they get to the far end of the bridge, the first part is already peeling and rusting. So they go back to the beginning to scrape and paint their way across the bridge again. It's an endless job; they never stop scraping and painting. Fresh paint is applied to the bridge as the old paint flakes off. The painters put on just enough paint to keep up with what comes off.

The amino acids in dietary protein are applied to the body in much the same way. Fresh amino acids come in after every meal, while the breakdown of tissue sloughs off old amino acids between meals. Like waves on a beach, there is a constant flux of old amino acids out, fresh amino acids in. The fresh amino acids grow new hair, skin, and all body tissues. The amino acids are available to all the organs, like fresh paint, to refurbish whatever structures are coming apart.

Apparently, on the Golden Gate Bridge, it does no good to hire more painters to put on more paint. The metal sloughs off the paint, thick or thin, in its own time. Similarly, it does no good to eat extra amino acids because the body uses only what it needs, wasting any extra.

Our analogy with the bridge breaks down on one point — the painters do not save and reuse the old, scraped-off paint. The body, however, can save and reuse a portion of its "old" amino acids. All of these amino acids, new and some of the old, are mixed together in what is called the amino acid pool, which is available for use throughout the body.

Using amino acids to construct new tissue can be compared to building a backyard shed. Picture a lumber truck pulling up to your house with a load of two by fours. The driver says, "I'll be back in a couple of hours." He didn't bring enough lumber to complete the project, so you decide to delay construction until he returns. A couple of hours later the truck pulls up to your house. The driver dumps some more lumber, then loads up all the two by fours he dumped before and leaves! "I'll be back in a couple of hours," he yells. "Wow!" you think, "I'd better use as much of that lumber as I can so he won't take it away the next time he comes!"

The process of tissue growth and repair is like that. The muscles can't stockpile their amino acids. They flow in right after a meal, but after a couple of hours, any that haven't been used are sucked right back out again. If we haven't eaten in a long time, the supply of new amino acids diminishes, and those in the tissues are "scraped" out, resulting in a net loss of tissue protein. Like the Golden Gate Bridge, we need fresh paint — fresh amino acids — continually to keep up with their ongoing loss.

Amino acids have another function beyond the building of tissues — sometimes they are converted into substitute sugar to be used as fuel for muscles or brain. It doesn't seem right to use amino acids intended for tissue repair simply as a fuel. That's as silly as burning expensive two by fours in your fireplace instead of a cheaper, more easily available fuel. But if the muscles and brain are not getting enough carbohydrate or fat fuel, the liver has to convert some amino acids into fuel.

Stress — emotional or physical — also triggers the liver to convert amino acids into glucose. The body says, "Oh-oh! this is an emergency. I may need more sugar." Stressor hormones are released that decrease the amount of amino acids entering muscle, forcing the amino acid pool to be available only to the liver. You can see why people under constant stress do not refurbish tissues or maintain healthy defenses. There is a direct link between stress and sickness.

"Does fasting cleanse the body?"

Fasting is also a "stress." Proponents claim that fasting cleanses the body. In one sense, they are quite right. Fasting does cleanse the body, but it doesn't clean out all those unnamed toxins they've dreamed up. Instead, fasting cleans out all the amino acids. If you don't eat, the amino acid pool is diminished, robbing tissues of their ability to repair.

You may conclude from all this that you need to eat extra protein, but as the two prior chapters have pointed out, most diets have more than enough protein. And as this chapter has pointed out, the body cannot use or stockpile extra amino acids anyway. The trick is to eat complex carbohydrates, thus providing a constant trickle of glucose energy and saving protein for growth and repair.

How Do Muscles Grow?

Let's compare muscle to a carpet factory. The factory has big machines to do the hard work and employees to run those big machines. The machines are impressive, but nothing would happen without the employees.

In muscle, the employees are ATP, creatine-P, sugar- and fat-burning enzymes, and Krebs-cycle enzymes. These protein chemicals run around moving energy and supplies where needed. But the actual work of contraction in muscle, the big machines, comes from an altogether different set of proteins called actin and myosin, together called actomyosin.

Long-distance runners are sometimes very skinny. They don't have large muscles or great lifting strength. They have developed their "employee" enzymes but not their actomyosin "machines." In contrast, some power weightlifters have big muscles from the growth of actomyosin, but they can't run well because they haven't increased their enzymes.

Suppose we wanted our carpet factory to produce more carpet. We could buy bigger, better machines, keep the same number of employees, and produce lots of carpet fast. But we'd have to shut down on weekends because our employees would be tired. That compares with weightlifting. Bigger muscles give more power, but they tire quickly.

We could take the opposite approach — increase the number of employees while using the same machines. Now our factory can operate three shifts, seven days a week, to produce more carpet. That is like endurance sports, which don't change the size of muscles but give them lasting energy.

Throughout this book we've talked about ways to increase the "employees" — enzymes — of muscle work. Now let's look at what makes the actual "machines" get bigger.

Actomyosin gives form and structure to muscle. The enlargement of muscle produced by weightlifting represents changes in actomyosin. Muscle enlargement, or hypertrophy, very much depends on working the muscle to maximum or near-maximum contraction. It's the *intensity* of contraction that stimulates hypertrophy more than the number of times it is contracted. Only a few maximal or near-maximal contractions a day are necessary for muscle growth. Many an overzealous bodybuilder finds that his muscles are getting smaller instead of larger because he's doing too many contractions or doing them too often.

> **Get rid of the piddly dumbbells.**
> **Hard muscles demand heavy iron.**

Make the muscle work hard and intensely and then let it rest. By rest I don't mean just the immediate rest you give the muscle between contractions but also the rest from one workout to the next. The classic rule is to rest a muscle for forty-eight hours between workouts. Some bodybuilders work out every day, but they don't work the same muscle group every day. It is during the resting period that new protein is synthesized, actomyosin grows, and the muscle gets larger.

Contraction alone is the essential stimulus necessary for muscle growth. We used to think that men's muscles hypertrophied more readily than women's because they have more testosterone. Scientists now believe that testosterone plays a limited role. At puberty it is responsible for making not only more fibers but also larger fibers. However, hypertrophy of these fibers seems to be independent of testosterone. A muscle fiber enlarges in response to one thing — demand. If it's contracted hard enough and often enough, it will get bigger. It will get bigger without hormones. It will get bigger without protein in the diet. It will even get bigger, for a time, in a person who is starving. When a muscle is repeatedly forced to contract to its maximum, it gets preferential access to the amino acid pools and hogs all the available proteins for muscle synthesis.

Fast Twitch, Slow Twitch

If you poked around in the muscle cells in the thigh, you would find, to your surprise, that some of the cells had lots of sugar-burning enzymes while others had few sugar-burning enzymes but lots of fat-burning enzymes. Those cells that are predominantly sugar burners, called fast-twitch fibers, are used for fast, contractional sports. Fast-twitch fibers don't have endurance, but they have a lot of snap and a lot of power. Neighboring muscle cells that burn fatty acids predominantly, called slow-twitch fibers, are for endurance. You use them when you go for a long, long time without stopping.

As the names indicate, fast-twitch fibers contract quickly and forcefully when stimulated, while slow-twitch fibers have a slower contraction speed and less force. Fast-twitch fibers also tend to hypertrophy (enlarge) more readily, thus enhancing the shape of muscles. They are sort of the glory hounds of musculature. Their actions and appearance get all the "oohs" and "ahhs" from spectators. They like to bask in the limelight, leaving the everyday drudgery of muscle work to the slow-twitch fibers. "We get tired too easily," they whine. "Let the slow-twitch fibers do the boring stuff." So the slow-twitch fibers do most of the work of moving us from place to place. The fast-twitch join in only when extra power is needed.

We know that muscle is responsible for burning up to 90 percent of the calories we eat every day. Of the two fiber types, it's the slow-twitch, aerobic fibers that are the real calorie burners because they do the majority of the work. Even skeletal

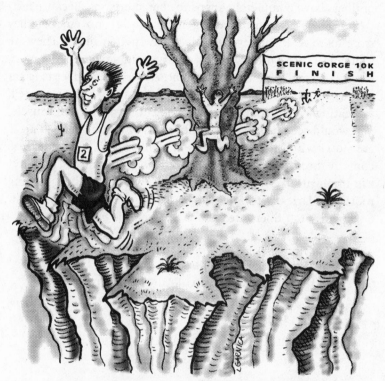

Joe seems to have an overabundance of fast-twitch muscles!

support, which we never think of as muscle work, is provided by the slow-twitch fibers. Your skeleton is just a pile of bones hooked together with ligaments. It's the slow-twitch fibers in muscles that hold them upright by providing constant, untiring tension.

Aerobic, slow-twitch fibers allow you to continue an activity for as long as fuel supplies are available. Slow-twitch fibers run marathons. Fast-twitch fibers go along for the marathon ride, waiting for the anaerobic sprint at the end.

The differences between fast-twitch and slow-twitch fibers are truly black and white. In every comparison the two kinds of fibers have completely opposite characteristics. Because fast-twitch fibers need instant energy for explosive movements, they store more ATP and glycogen than slow-twitch fibers. They are more elastic to protect against injury from sudden movement. The two even look entirely different. A fast-twitch fiber is larger and usually pale, while a slow-twitch is smaller and deep red, indicating a rich blood supply. If you cut across a fresh muscle, you would see areas of red next to areas of white. The red areas are slow-twitch fibers with lots of capillaries. The white areas contain the fast-twitch fibers with fewer capillaries. Think of the implications of this difference. Slow-twitch fibers, having more capillaries, get more oxygen, which is needed to burn fat. So slow-twitch fibers are the fat burners, the calorie users.

> **Fast-twitch fibers are the glory hounds of musculature, getting all the "oohs" and "ahhs" from spectators.**

More about Lactic Acid

Fast- and slow-twitch fibers interact in an interesting way in the production and use of lactic acid. When you pedal a bicycle uphill, the fast-twitch fibers usually produce lactic acid in the thigh muscles, and you feel the burn. The slow-twitch fibers, which work only when oxygen is present, have probably stopped. Once you're over the top of the hill and are pedaling easily down the other side, the burn goes away. That's because the lactic acid produced by the fast-twitch fibers trickles into the adjoining slow-twitch fibers, which metabolize it aerobically. In other words, lactic acid produced in a fast-twitch fiber as a waste product trickles over and is used by a slow-twitch fiber as a fuel source.

How is it possible for the lactic acid to be burned if there's no oxygen available? The answer is — not ALL of your cells are low in oxygen. The fast-twitch fibers, having few aerobic (oxidative) enzymes, make lactic acid easily, then call up their slow-twitch buddies. "Hey! We've got a lot of lactic acid building up in here. Can we send it over to you guys?" The slow-twitch fibers reply, "Sure thing! Our oxidative enzymes are working just fine." The lactate is shipped either directly or via the bloodstream. The slow-twitch fibers don't seem to care whether their fuel is glucose or lactic acid. Either one works fine for them.

This explains why the best way to get rid of the burn is to keep exercising at a slower pace. Lactic acid is eliminated much more quickly during walking than during complete rest. If you cool down rather than sit down, blood continues to flow rapidly through your muscles. This higher rate of blood flow helps transport lactate to all those tissues in the body that have plenty of oxidative enzymes and are hungry for some fuel to burn.

> **"What's the best way to get rid of the burn?"**

Getting the burn now and then actually improves aerobic fitness. Theoretically, gentle, lactic-acid-avoiding exercise will eventually get you fit. But that's not the most up-to-date advice. Some intense exercise, such as the wind sprints I described before, interspersed in an aerobic workout raises fitness much more quickly. People who want to be very fit, up in the competition range, find that they must include some lactic-acid-producing sprint activity in their training. Even if their competition sport is an aerobic one such as marathoning or bicycling, they need to do something anaerobic if they want to get fitter.

Of course, the more aerobically trained you are, the less often you will experience the burn. Aerobically fit muscles have lots of oxidative enzymes to process the lactate produced, so you can exercise longer and harder before you get the burn. People who cross-train have the same advantage. The more total muscle trained, the better chance of processing lactic acid.

Do Men Have More Fast-Twitch Fibers?

An average person's total musculature is about 50 percent fast-twitch and 50 percent slow-twitch fibers, although in specific muscles one type usually predominates. The muscles of the calf, for example, are predominantly fast-twitch fibers so that you can sprint when necessary, but they also contain slow-twitch fibers so you can walk for miles without getting tired. Likewise the biceps and triceps have a higher proportion of fast-twitch fibers for quick and powerful movements such as throwing or jumping. The muscles of the thighs, hips, and back have more slow-twitch fibers, which provide tension for posture and stamina for endurance activities. The heart muscle is almost totally slow-twitch because it's an endurance muscle. The heart has a higher concentration of aerobic, fatty-acid-burning enzymes than any other muscle. Aerobic exercise builds in other muscles those same aerobic capabilities — it's as if skeletal muscles wanted to emulate the heart muscle.

The 50 percent fast-twitch and 50 percent slow-twitch mixture applies to sedentary people. Athletes tend to have more of one type or the other, depending on their sport. We usually see more slow-twitch fibers in men and women trained for endurance sports, while the sprinting and power-sport athletes tend to have more fast-twitch fibers. In the next chapter I'll take a look at the possible explanations for these variations.

What about male and female muscle? Since men have bigger

muscles than women, do they have more fast-twitch fibers? Yes, they do, but not proportionately more; that is, they also have more slow-twitch fibers, so the comparative percentages remain the same. Sedentary men have the same fiber distribution as sedentary women, while athletic men and women have slightly higher percentages of one or the other, depending on their sport.

> **Women can "bulk up" as easily as men.**

Men also have larger muscle fibers. These two factors — larger fibers and more numerous fibers — have led to the misconception that men "bulk up" more easily than women. However, recent studies show that male and female muscle hypertrophies, or bulks up, equally well. If men and women lift weights for the same number of repetitions at the same relative intensity (women lift lighter weights since their muscles are smaller), the percentage of enlargement is nearly identical for both sexes. In one study, for example, men and women did biceps curls for sixteen weeks. After the maximum amount of weight they could curl was determined, they did as many repetitions as possible at 70–90 percent of that maximum on three alternate days a week. At the end of sixteen weeks, both the men and the women had about a 7 percent increase in arm circumference.

The men appeared to get bigger than the women because they had more muscle to start with. A 7 percent enlargement in a little arm doesn't appear as significant as a 7 percent enlargement in a big arm. Men have an advantage because the testosterone produced during puberty gives them more and bigger fibers. But after puberty those fibers do not appear to require testosterone. A fast-twitch fiber, be it male or female, hypertrophies in response to demand.

Does the Type of Training Determine Fiber Type?

Muscle fibers are the classic example of the adage "form follows function." Whatever type of training you do, the fiber will enhance its characteristics to oblige you. Lots of long-distance training increases the fat-burning enzymes in the slow-twitch fibers. Weightlifting or sprinting builds the sugar-burning enzymes inside the fast-twitch fibers while also increasing the size of the fibers.

What about the fibers themselves? Do different kinds of training change the proportion of slow- and fast-twitch fibers? We know that people who compete in endurance sports such as cycling and running tend to have a higher percentage of slow-twitch fibers (around 63 percent) compared to sedentary people (48 percent). Similarly, power lifters have a higher percentage of fast-twitch fibers than the average person. The question for both endurance and power athletes is, do they have more slow-twitch or fast-twitch fibers because their training increased that type of fiber? Or did they succeed in their sport because they were born with a higher percentage of that fiber, while other athletes, with lower percentages, were weeded out? In other words, does training or heredity account for a predominance of fiber type?

Several studies on twins have tended to support the latter argument; that is, you're born with a certain number of fast-twitch or slow-twitch fibers, and nothing you do later can change it. These studies show that identical twins (developed from the same egg and therefore having the same genetic makeup) have the same proportion of fast- and slow-twitch fibers even though one twin is active in endurance sports while the other does power sports. The power-sports twin may have *larger* fast-twitch fibers (a "form follows function" adaptation) than the endurance-sport twin, but both have the *same percentage* of the two fiber types. These studies seem to support the dictum that the body makes a fixed number of muscle cells. What you're born with, you're stuck with. The cells can enlarge or shrink, but you don't get more of them.

> **"Do endurance athletes have more slow-twitch fibers because of their training — or were they born with them?"**

However, recent studies offer a possible contradiction. Some animal studies have shown an actual increase in the number of fibers, not just their size, in response to heavy resistance training. Also, athletes who rely on both endurance and power, such as swimmers and kayakers, display enlarged deltoids even though the diameter of their muscle fibers is surprisingly small. If the fibers didn't enlarge but the overall muscle size did, it *may* be that the number of fibers increased.

The data on the numbers-versus-size argument are not yet conclusive, and most researchers tend to stick with "you can change the size of the fiber but you can't change the number of fibers."

Can You Switch Your Twitch?

Since most research says that training does not increase the *number* of muscle fibers, is it possible to change the characteristics of existing fibers? Wouldn't it be neat if we could change some of our fast-twitch fibers into fat-burning, calorie-consuming, fatigue-resistant slow-twitch fibers? The answer, incredibly, is that we can — by surgically changing the nerve supply to the fiber. Of course it's only been done on animals, but let me describe the basis for the procedure. It has some interesting similarities to aerobic exercise.

The characteristics of a muscle are determined by the nerve supplying it. A single nerve controls several muscle fibers to form what is called a motor unit. Some motor units, such as the abdominals, consist of hundreds of fibers controlled by a single nerve, while others, like the muscles of the eyes, have as few as ten fibers supplied by one nerve. The fibers of a motor unit are always either fast-twitch or slow-twitch, even though they may be surrounded by motor units that have the opposite characteristics.

Thus the muscles of the calf can be a mixture of slow-twitch and fast-twitch because different nerves innervate the various individual fibers. The nerve programs the fiber to contract quickly or more slowly. It also determines whether the fiber has more sugar-burning or more fat-burning enzymes. I realize that this may sound confusing, but in a nutshell, the nerve determines fiber type and function.

Researchers can surgically switch the nerves to muscle fibers (called cross-innervation) and change one fiber type to the other. An interesting thing about these experiments is that the fiber changes in an orderly sequence. If, for instance, the nerve to a fast-twitch fiber is replaced with a nerve for slow-twitch fibers, the fast-twitch fiber will first start making more fat-burning enzymes. Then more capillaries slowly appear in and around the fiber. Next the sugar-burning enzymes diminish so that the fiber contracts more slowly. Finally, the composition of the protein in the fiber wall changes. Talk about the adaptability of muscle! In an almost magical way, that fast-twitch fiber now looks, contracts, and functions like a slow-twitch fiber.

Interesting as that may be, surgically switching nerves doesn't seem to be a practical solution to producing more slow-twitch, fat-burning fibers. Well, there's another way to do it. If you attach an electrode to the nerve and run a low, continuous current through it, the fiber goes through all those same orderly changes. You don't like this idea either? There is a third method, but so far researchers have demonstrated it only in rabbits, rats, and other small rodents. It's called exercise. Very, very long exercise seems to mimic the stimulation to the nerve that an electrical current provides. When rats are made to run uphill three to four hours a day for several months, some of their fast-twitch fibers make the full conversion into slow-twitch fibers.

Can the same thing happen in humans who train extraordinarily long and hard? There isn't enough research to know for sure, primarily because the testing takes too long. In rats, significant changes are evident in weeks or months, but it may take years for the same changes to show up in humans.

Even though it hasn't been proven, it's still interesting to speculate why elite endurance athletes have such a high percentage of slow-twitch fibers. Were they born with them, or is it possible that years and years of endurance activity have caused some of their fast-twitch fibers to gradually change?

Consider also the exercise-induced muscle changes seen in any endurance athlete. More capillaries grow to deliver oxygen to the muscle, and the fat-burning enzymes increase. These enzyme and capillary changes are identical to the initial changes that occur when a fast-twitch muscle fiber is converting to a slow-twitch fiber by cross-innervation or electrical stimulation.

So! The answer to the question of whether you can change fiber type is uncertain at this time. Perhaps in humans, only the initial changes are possible. However, we know this for certain — endurance exercise enhances the characteristics of existing slow-twitch fibers. They grow more fat-burning enzymes, they develop more capillaries, and they learn to function for longer and longer periods without fatigue.

> **Having more slow-twitch fibers is appealing because they are the butter-burning fibers.**

Having more slow-twitch fibers or slow-twitch characteristics is, of course, appealing, since these are the butter-burning fibers. But don't despair if you lean toward being a fast-twitch type. Those born with predominantly fast-twitch muscles have an advantage. They can participate more easily in the quick, explosive sports, but they can also switch to long-distance, slow-twitch sports if they train long and hard enough. In contrast, those born with slow-twitch muscles must stick with endurance sports.

The Fat Weightlifter

For weightlifters the drawback to bigger muscles is that there is no accompanying increase in capillaries. The muscle doesn't lose capillaries, but new ones don't grow to nourish the added bulk, so there are fewer capillaries per square inch. Additionally, muscles that have enlarged from weightlifting have proportionately fewer fat-burning enzymes. While they're great for explosive or power moves, hypertrophied muscles often lack long-term endurance. This explains why many power lifters do poorly on fitness tests. Despite their muscle mass, they have limited capacity for sustained exercise. This also explains why power lifters tend to be fat. Anaerobic, sugar-burning activity does not burn fat. Aerobic activity does.

"But," you argue, "I know lots of bodybuilders who are not fat!" We need to make a distinction here between power lifters and bodybuilders. When I talk about power lifters, I'm referring to the Olympic-type lifters. When they train, they lift very heavy weights very few times. This kind of high-intensity training means that their muscles rely largely on the creatine-P system for energy. Very little of their glycogen or fat is used during such workouts. This also means that little fat is needed *after* their workout to replace glycogen.

Bodybuilders follow a different program. Their workouts involve slightly lighter weights with more repetitions. Their training also includes running, cycling, or other aerobic exercise. Their workouts use more of the lactate and aerobic systems. As you recall, fat is burned only in the aerobic system, but both systems drain the muscles of glycogen, which then has to be replaced following exercise. Replacing glycogen requires burning fat, so the bodybuilder gets the best of two worlds. He gets the muscle enlargement and strength associated with sugar-burning sports and the oxidative enzyme growth and new capillaries associated with endurance sports. Also most bodybuilders are quite strict about the amount of fat in their diet. Added together, these three things — weightlifting, aerobic exercise, and careful dieting — make for very attractive, highly muscled, low-fat bodies.

> **Power lifters often do poorly on fitness tests.**

The title of the chapter was intended to make weightlifters mad enough to read the chapter. Having read it, you can see through my trickery. The only weightlifters who are fat are those who do zero aerobic endurance exercise, lift the heaviest possible weights only two to three repetitions, and eat lots of fat-filled protein.

Anabolic Steroids

Anabolic steroids were first used in the 1940s on concentration camp survivors to rebuild muscle after the ravages of severe malnutrition. Then athletes got wind of the muscle-enhancing capabilities of the new drugs. They used the artificial steroids so much in the 1950s and '60s that scientists decided to test the drugs to see if they really worked. The scientists concluded that taking steroids did not enhance athletic performance. Bodybuilders and track-and-field athletes shook their heads in disbelief. "Look at us!" they exclaimed. "We're stronger, we run faster, our muscles are bigger. Of course steroids work!"

It turns out that nonathletes were used for the studies. In a nonathlete, steroids go to the muscles and say, "Do you need us?" "Naw," the muscles answer, "he isn't doing anything. Why don't you just go liven up his libido for a while?" The researchers concluded that since these nonathletes weren't any stronger or bigger, steroids were useless. Athletes, on the other hand, concluded that the researchers were useless. We now know that steroids not only help rebuild severely wasted muscles, they also enlarge and strengthen normal muscles — IF the muscles are worked hard.

So now doctors are saying, "Okay, we were wrong. Steroids do work, but you shouldn't take them because they're dangerous." Athletes compare their beautifully sculpted physiques to the pear shape of some myopic researcher and conclude that the doctors don't know anything.

Let's put the cards on the table. There is no doubt that steroids enhance strength and performance in practicing athletes. There is also no doubt that steroids are intertwined with practically every body function. Athletes have experienced the positive effects of steroids. Medical people have seen the dangerous effects of steroid imbalance. They know that when you tamper with the body's natural balance of steroids — testosterone, estrogen, or cortisone, for example — you are playing with fire.

Steroids are hormones secreted by various glands, in much the same way that spit is secreted by the salivary glands. Steroids and other hormones, however, are secreted directly into the blood, eventually reaching every tissue and organ. Each hormone has a specific action, and the body must make sure that one hormone does not duplicate or interfere with the action of another. So each one is equipped with "keys" that open certain cell doors but not others. The hormone called insulin, for instance, has a key that can open up cell walls so that blood glucose can get into the cell. If a person is insulin deficient (has diabetes), her cells don't unlock and sugar builds up in the bloodstream.

In a similar manner, parathormone from the parathyroid glands regulates the level of calcium in the blood. When blood calcium gets too low, the parathyroids produce more hormone, which then travels to the bones and "unlocks" the stored calcium. The bones release calcium into the blood until the proper level is reached.

A study of the function of all the hormones would take an entire book. They monitor mineral and fluid levels, control metabolism, and program development. Too much or too little of a single hormone can have a devastating effect on the whole body, as evidenced in dwarfs and giants, diabetics, cretins, and even in some obese people.

To guard against hormone malfunction, the pituitary gland at the base of the brain produces hormones that control the production of other hormones. The body also has the ability to partially convert one hormone into another. Excess quantities of estrogen can be converted into testosterone and vice versa.

Cortisone, aldosterone, estrogen, progesterone, testosterone, and forty other hormones that regulate everything from the amount of water in the body to sexuality can be partially interconverted. The amount of one hormone greatly influences the amounts of others. That is why our medical people were so scared of the first birth control pills, which are based on estrogen. And, if you recall, the pills did produce a host of side effects, including blood clots.

> **Hormone balance is an extremely delicate seesaw that is easily thrown off by random additional hormones.**

Even hydrocortisone injections, useful as they are for tennis elbow and bursitis, can potentially upset delicate hormone balances. Once I strained my shoulder paddling my canoe too long and too hard. Putting on a T-shirt by myself was almost impossible because I couldn't lift my arm. I knew and my doctor knew that one shot of hydrocortisone into the shoulder muscle could eliminate the problem. But we were afraid that some hydrocortisone might get into the blood and influence the delicate balance of other similar compounds, so we tried other treatments first.

The body's regulation of hormones is an extremely delicate seesaw that is easily thrown off by any randomly added hormones. Anabolic steroids are synthetic derivatives of the male hormone testosterone. Apparently they affect the pituitary somewhat like the real thing. When the pituitary senses a rise in anabolic steroids, it reacts just as if the level of testosterone were rising. It sends a message to the testes and the adrenal glands saying, "Okay, boys, you can shut down now. There's enough testosterone circulating." But macho Bill keeps taking the drug, and the pituitary starts to get worried. "A joke's a joke, guys. Slow it down. He's got acne, his hair is greasy, and he's starting to get belligerent." But the steroid level continues to rise. "All right, I've had it with you!" the pituitary warns. "If you don't cut this out, I'm going to shrivel up his testicles!"

That happens, in fact, in rats that have been given large doses of steroids. In humans who take steroids, natural testosterone levels decrease dramatically and remain low for weeks after the steroids are discontinued. In some cases, testosterone production never goes back to normal, resulting in permanent sterility.

If you don't believe that such drastic results can happen, talk to some of the women who were the first users of the birth control pill. Back then the hormones in the pill weren't properly balanced, and some longtime users were never able to get pregnant even after they stopped taking it.

Steroids are fantastically powerful and do have their place in medicine. After a month of other treatments that were ineffectual, my shoulder responded completely and totally to one shot of hydrocortisone. Used properly, steroids can do miracles. However, anabolic steroids are obtained on the black market, and there are no controls on their content, purity, or dosage. There is no telling what kind of damage they can cause, especially in a teenager who is already going through some pretty dramatic hormone changes. Of particular concern is that many athletes like to "stack" the drugs; that is, they take three or four different kinds of steroids simultaneously to really trigger the muscle-building effect.

Research is scanty. Experimenting with anabolic steroids on human subjects is considered unethical and dangerous. Therefore many of the warnings to date come from rat studies or from conjecture and hearsay. We hear that a football star taking steroids has a stroke and dies at the age of twenty-nine. Or a bodybuilder gets liver cancer after taking steroids for years. Or a steroid-using basketball player gets "roid rage" and beats up his girlfriend. Cancer, heart disease, psychosis — all have been linked to steroid use, but data are scarce.

What isn't scarce are studies linking steroids with changes in

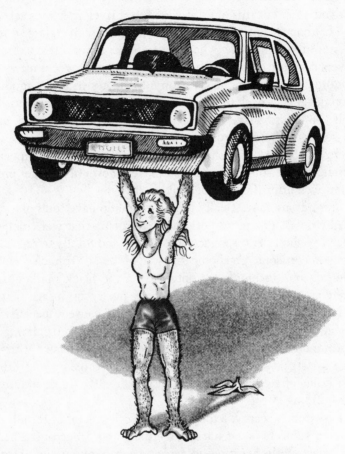

Margaret notices unusual
developments since taking steroids.

blood cholesterol. In general, people who are sedentary or obese or who smoke have low levels of the "good" cholesterol, high-density lipoprotein; low levels of HDL are associated with a higher incidence of atherosclerosis, heart attack, and stroke. Athletes, on the other hand, ordinarily have high HDL readings *unless* they take anabolic steroids. HDL levels are 50 percent lower in steroid-using athletes than in other athletes. This effect is seen even in women, who characteristically have high HDL levels until menopause. For those who like numbers:

	ATHLETES WHO USE STEROIDS		ATHLETES WHO DO NOT USE STEROIDS	
	Total cholesterol (mg/100 ml)	*HDL (mg/100 ml)*	*Total cholesterol (mg/100 ml)*	*HDL (mg/100 ml)*
Male	291	23.5	183	52.0
Female	216	30.6	173	66.2

One might argue that if we compared a steroid user to an average person instead of to highly trained athletes, the cholesterol levels would probably be about the same. Nope. Not only are cholesterol levels of steroid users bad when compared to the average person, they're bad when compared to people with an established high risk of heart disease:

	HIGH-RISK POPULATION	
	Total cholesterol (mg/100 ml)	*HDL (mg/100 ml)*
Male	221	43.7
Female	214	45.6

These data aren't from an isolated study or a small population. The research has been duplicated over and over. I sure hope it scares any of my readers who are thinking of taking steroids.

One problem with anabolic steroids is that manufacturers cannot completely get rid of the masculine side effects. For a man, this is no big deal, but what if you're a female bodybuilder taking steroids to be more muscular than other women? Pretty soon you're shaving a little mustache every day, you sound like a stevedore, and you're getting mighty feisty with your friends. Steroid users say the effects wear off after they stop taking the drug, but enlargement of the larynx (which deepens the voice) and the loss of scalp hair are irreversible in women.

12

The Payoff

*You could replace all the good information
in this book with vigorous sport.
Just get involved, and the benefits
will roll in automatically!*

Exercise and Blood Pressure

Exercise and Cholesterol

Stress

Decreasing the Risk of Heart Attacks

The Hollow-Leg Syndrome

Are You a Mercedes or a Pinto?

Exercise and Blood Pressure

If blood volume rises as a result of exercise, it seems that blood pressure should also rise, just as the pressure rises in a hose if you turn up the flow of water. But it doesn't! Fit people actually have lower blood pressure both at rest and during exercise. To understand why, let's compare the blood system to a hose attached to a shower head that delivers water in spurts instead of a steady flow. It can pump small spurts of water quickly or large spurts more slowly. In each case the total output is the same. A sedentary person's heart pumps quickly, but not much blood is pumped with each stroke. A fit person's heart pumps a larger volume per contraction but contracts fewer times per minute. As above, in each case the total cardiac output is the same.

Now suppose the faucet is turned up so that it spurts very rapidly *and* lots of water is pumped with each spurt. The pressure in the hose is going to rise. The same thing happens in the blood vessels of both fit and unfit people. You'd think that it would rise really high in fit people since they have a greater volume of blood, but it doesn't because they also have more capillaries in their muscles. If the blood can "escape" into hundreds and hundreds of capillaries (which also, by the way, enlarge with exercise), then overall pressure is reduced.

It used to be common to hear that every extra pound of fat requires miles of extra capillaries and therefore means more work for the heart. You can see the falsehood of this statement because more capillaries means reduced pressure and *less* work for the heart. The original claim is wrong. Fat people have high blood pressure because their unused muscle has fewer capillaries. If a fat, hypertensive person begins a regular exercise routine, his blood pressure decreases as he gets fit even if his weight stays the same.

> **Blood pressure often decreases in a fat person who exercises — even if he doesn't lose weight.**

These two factors, lowered heart rate and increased capillarity, explain why regular exercise actually lowers blood pressure rather than raising it. The more consistent the exercise, the more effectively it lowers blood pressure. Studies have shown that thirty-minute sessions of mild aerobic exercise (60–70 percent maximum heart rate) cause blood pressure to drop immediately after the exercise, and significantly lower pressure persists on subsequent nonexercise days. If you exercise on a regular schedule, you can lower your blood pressure consistently.

To be most effective, the exercise should involve a lot of muscle. The more muscles used at one time, the better. When large masses of muscle are worked, more and more capillaries open up, allowing the blood to "spread out" so that the overall pressure is lowered. Some kinds of aerobic exercise are more effective than others. Stationary bicycling uses relatively few muscles, mainly the quadriceps, and it therefore doesn't have as much effect on blood pressure as jogging. The emphasis here is not how hard or intense the exercise but how many muscles are involved. Vigorous walking or gentle jogging causes more capillaries to dilate, even though these exercises are less intense than pedaling furiously on a stationary bicycle.

Weightlifting, even though it uses lots of muscles, doesn't lower blood pressure because each individual lift uses only a few muscles intensely. The vessels to the muscle group being worked dilate, but the vessels to the rest of the body constrict.

The proportion of dilated vessels is much smaller than the proportion of contracted vessels, so overall blood pressure actually rises during high-intensity weight training.

Does this mean you shouldn't lift if you have high blood pressure? Most physicians say that people with moderate or severe high blood pressure should not lift weights. If hypertension is mild, researchers have found that low-intensity circuit training with high repetitions and low weights (40 percent of maximum ability) is safe and may even help lower blood pressure. People who teach circuit training love to quote these researchers, but there's really nothing special about this information. The more "aerobic" the weight training, the more it approaches systemic exercise; that is, the more the weight training deviates from classic high-weight, low-rep lifting, the more effective it will be in controlling blood pressure.

Mild hypertension can usually be lowered by exercise alone, making drugs unnecessary. However, if you do have high blood pressure that must be controlled with drugs, let your physician know that you exercise regularly. He can then experiment to see which type of drug interferes least with your exercise. Some of the beta blockers impair exercise performance and interfere with the dissipation of heat, so they are not favored by athletes. Also, you and your physician will have to consider whether the use of diuretics is warranted. These are often prescribed for hypertension to help get rid of excess water, but they may exacerbate dehydration during exercise. Another thing to consider is that some antihypertensive drugs make you retain more potassium. Athletes often take aspirin, nonsteroid anti-inflammatory medications, or even sports drinks that contain potassium, and all of these can magnify the potassium-retaining effects of the high blood pressure medication.

Exercise and Cholesterol

Cholesterol is a fat! Fats don't mix with water! To get cholesterol to dissolve in watery blood, the liver wraps it with some protein so that the blood won't see it as a fat. When the protein wrapping is heavy and thick, the cholesterol is called high-density lipoprotein or HDL. When it is rather thin, it is called low-density lipoprotein or LDL.

In the past, physicians were concerned only with the total level of cholesterol in the blood. Nowadays they also want to know the levels of HDL and LDL. A high level of HDL is a sign of good health, so HDL has become the "good cholesterol."

Although we hear the terms often, it isn't really fair to say that LDL is bad and HDL is good. Cholesterol is simply transported in the bloodstream in different forms. The "bad" form, LDL, is actually the more common means of transport, accounting for almost three-quarters of all blood cholesterol. If most of the cholesterol is transported by the "bad" method, then there must be a "good" reason for it!

When the liver wants to send a bunch of triglycerides to fat depots, it wraps them in a thin layer of protein — LDL. The protein is really fragile because the triglycerides need to escape easily when they reach the depots. Even though triglycerides are the main item being transported, some cholesterol tags along for the ride. After the triglycerides are released, the cholesterol is left behind. Unfortunately, the thin protein coating is not strong enough to contain the cholesterol, which then gets dumped off in all the wrong places — such as the lining of arteries.

When you realize the purpose of low-density lipoprotein — to transport triglycerides to fat-storage facilities — you see why it is made. It comes apart easily so that the triglycerides can get into fat cells. But too much LDL is a problem in that it tends to deposit cholesterol in the arteries. LDL in itself is not bad unless there's too much of it or it isn't balanced by a healthy amount of HDL.

The heavier wrapping on HDL makes sure the cholesterol goes to its intended destination, where it is used properly. People think cholesterol is a horrible thing, but it is a key ingredient in bile; without it we wouldn't be able to digest fat. Without cholesterol we wouldn't have male or female characteristics, because it is a component of the steroid hormones. For that matter, we wouldn't even exist, since cholesterol is a major constituent of all cell membranes.

> **Aerobic exercise may not lower your total blood cholesterol, but it sure raises the "good guys"!**

En route to its final destination, HDL has a neat way of cleaning the arteries by picking up cholesterol from them. It gets its "good" reputation because it *may* actually remove cholesterol from plaque deposits on coronary artery walls. In proper balance, HDL and LDL are neither good nor bad. They simply have two different delivery systems. It's when they get out of balance that problems arise. HDL and LDL are balanced when HDL comprises at least 25 percent of total cholesterol.

Endurance exercise significantly raises the level of HDL. Fit people have "fit" livers that cover cholesterol with extra protein. Endurance exercise also seems to lower the total level of cholesterol, but we don't know if it's the exercise itself that causes this or other changes associated with exercise, in particular, weight loss.

To raise your HDL cholesterol, you have to exercise at aerobic intensity (65 to 80 percent of maximum heart rate) and you have to do it thirty to forty minutes a day, three to four days a week. Sadly, many people with high cholesterol are fat or out of shape, and they find exercise unappealing. If you're one of these people, don't be discouraged. Studies have shown that the more unfit you are, the more significant your improvement will be. It requires an intense amount of exercise for very fit people to get even small changes in their HDL, but very unfit people get major changes quickly. They don't have to run marathons. If even three exercise sessions a week seems daunting, just go for a walk or play some golf. While these low-intensity activities don't affect HDL, they *have* been shown to lower total cholesterol and LDL. It's true that more vigorous, aerobic activity is necessary to raise your HDL, but by starting with the easy stuff, like walking, the good changes you see may encourage you to try the harder stuff later.

Stress

When we're in stressful situations, our adrenal glands secrete special hormones to help us through the stress. These hormones include epinephrine (also called adrenaline), norepinephrine, and cortisol. They prepare our bodies to handle stress by speeding up the heart rate to increase cardiac output, constricting the blood vessels to the gut while enlarging those to the muscles, and dilating the pupils to give us a better look at whatever we're confronting. They stimulate the liver to release its glucose stores for quick energy. Fat depots are induced to liberate free fatty acids for fuel. The release of stress hormones produces a heightened state of awareness that helps us think more clearly and quickly.

The good thing about these hormones is that they prepare the body to run away from danger. The stress response is quite fabulous — it's pulled a lot of people through situations that would otherwise have killed them. The problem is that when the stress is emotional, the same array of physiological changes occurs, and if you pile on enough emotional stress, the system works against you rather than for you.

Just the rerouting of amino acids, for example, is enough to cause problems. Amino acids are supposed to be used for tissue growth and repair, but when you are under constant emotional stress, they are removed from tissues and burned for flight fuel instead. That's why many people lose weight when they are under stress for a long time. Their muscles waste away as the repair and growth of new tissue slacks off.

The production of antibodies from amino acids also diminishes, making the immune system less hardy. Invading bacteria from a cut are less likely to be mopped up by the white blood cells. Stressed people get sick more easily as viruses sneak into unprotected tissues.

What we need is a drug that will encourage our adrenal glands to secrete more stress hormones when we really need them for physical stresses and fewer hormones when we are emotionally stressed. You will be pleased to know that such a drug is available; it's called exercise.

Extensive studies on rats and baboons have shown that when they are exposed to mild but repeated stress such as cold, shock treatment, restraint, intermittent loud noises, or aerobic exercise, there is a big change in their stress responses. They get tough, able to handle the stress better. And they handle it better in two ways. First, if the stress is something with which they are familiar, they produce smaller amounts of stress hormones. It's as if their bodies say, "Ho-hum. We're used to that stress. We don't have to get in a snit over it." Second, if the stressful situation is novel, something they haven't previously experienced, they produce more stress hormones than normal. Their bodies gear up better than usual to cope with the stress. Additionally, after the stress is over, their bodies are able to get rid of the no-longer-needed hormones faster.

> **Aerobic exercise is a stress that makes us tough enough to handle all other stresses.**

Humans don't "volunteer" for these kinds of experiments as readily as rats. The only stress we routinely submit to is aerobic exercise. And it's been shown that very fit, aerobically trained people, like stressed rats, have a diminished response to everyday stresses yet a heightened response to novel situations.

When you start an aerobic exercise program, the adrenals secrete lots of stress hormones, but after a couple of months, they produce much less even though you're doing the same amount of work. As your tissues become more sensitive to the hormones, you get the same response from less stimulation. As the saying goes, a little bit (of stressor hormones) now goes a long way. The effect spills over into other parts of your life, so everyday problems don't evoke typical stress reactions. If you're pushing to meet a deadline at work, you won't be as stressed out if you're aerobically fit. If your kids are screaming, the soup is burning on the stove, and the cat is sampling your bridge party's hors d'oeuvres, you'll handle it better if you've been jogging regularly. Your blood pressure won't rise, you'll feel calmer, and you'll have a sense of being able to cope. When we say that aerobic exercise helps us deal with stress, there's a very real physiological explanation for it. What is stressful to a sedentary person is less stressful to an exercised person.

The key point here is that adaptation to exercise also produces a mental adaptation. Highly fit people usually present three personality traits: they do well in stress/challenge tests, they exhibit emotional stability, and they are more resistant to depression and anxiety.

The beauty of aerobic conditioning is that when you need that extra adrenaline wallop, it's there. If you're fit, you'll produce more than the normal amounts of adrenal hormones when faced with a new, stressful situation. At rest, you'll have lower than normal stress hormone levels, but the level can "spike" when you're confronted with stress or challenge.

Decreasing the Risk
of Heart Attacks

By now you can probably see why exercise protects against heart disease. Many, many changes take place beyond improvements in your heart, lungs, and muscles. Exercise induces subtle changes in blood that in roundabout ways ease the work of the heart. Even the way blood coagulates in fit people helps to reduce their risk of heart attack.

After exercise, blood clots faster. Oddly, almost contradictorily, exercised blood also *unclots* faster. It's as if exercise puts the body into a heightened state of readiness. Exercise is a stress: your body doesn't know if you're running for the fun of it or because a bear is chasing you. It says, "Oh-oh. She's running! If something is chasing her, I'd better make sure she doesn't bleed to death if she gets caught. I'd better speed up the clotting mechanisms. But if she doesn't get caught, then I'd better make sure that the circulating blood doesn't turn into a whole bunch of clots." As a result, both the clotting and the anticlotting mechanisms are enhanced.

Clotting, or coagulation, is a fairly complicated process. It would take several pages to describe it, but essentially the body can make a clotting "bandage" that would put Johnson & Johnson to shame. It produces just enough clotting chemicals to make the right-sized bandage and then makes anticlotting chemicals to stop the bandage from getting too big. The balance between the clotting and anticlotting mechanisms is delicate. Exercise enhances both processes.

The balance is fairly even, but recent research indicates that in regular exercisers the balance may tilt slightly toward the anticlotting mechanisms. This is good because it means that regular activity can reduce the risk of heart attacks and strokes.

The underlying cause of heart disease is the buildup of fatty deposits (atherosclerotic plaques) inside blood vessels. But a heart attack usually occurs when a blood clot forms directly over these deposits and then breaks off, plugging a vessel. In 85 percent of cases a blood clot is the final event causing a heart attack or stroke. Most of the time the body naturally dissolves small clots before they break off, so you're never aware of anything being wrong.

> **Even though it takes years and years of exercise to strengthen the heart itself, its function improves immediately with aerobic exercise because of the many small changes elsewhere in the body that ease the work of the heart.**

A substance in the blood called plasminogen is converted into plasmin to help dissolve clots. To activate the plasminogen so that it becomes plasmin, the cells lining blood vessels produce a substance called tissue plasminogen activator (tPA). Wouldn't it be great if we could somehow make more tPA? Right — you've already figured it out. Fit people produce more tPA than unfit people. In a six-month program of moderate aerobic exercise, a group of people ranging from twenty to seventy-four years in age had an average increase in tPA of 29 percent. At the same time, one of the clotting factors found in blood, fibrinogen, decreased slightly. The implication here is that people who exercise may have a protective clot dissolver that sedentary people lack.

Exercised blood is different. It's thinner, so the heart doesn't have to work as hard. It has more red blood cells and thus a greater oxygen supply, so oxygen is delivered more efficiently. It has less fat so vessels don't get sludged up with plaques. It has hormones and neurotransmitters that relax those blood vessels. And exercised blood stimulates the production of substances that fight clots in those vessels.

All these subtle changes ease the work of the heart, decrease clotting in the blood vessels, and significantly lower the incidence of cardiovascular disease and heart attacks.

The Hollow-Leg Syndrome

Personally, I suspect that people who are extraordinarily fit have a lowered basal metabolism, not the higher basal metabolic rate that so many people claim. Picture a very fit man sitting next to a very out-of-shape man. Which one is more likely to be panting for air? Which has the faster heart rate? Very fit people breathe more slowly and have slower heart rates than unfit people, which probably indicates a lower basal metabolism. Well, if exercise does not increase the basal metabolism of very fit people and may in fact lower it, why don't they gain weight?

The answer, of course, is obvious. All the other metabolisms speed up. They tend to fidget more. Their bodies churn out heat like crazy. They digest enormous amounts of food. It doesn't matter how much they eat; they seem to have a hollow leg. The repair of tissues and resynthesis of energy stores is a never-ending process. And — they exercise ALL THE TIME!

Let's go back to my average woman and her graph in the chapter on metabolism (page 61). Male readers, please extrapolate a bit. My average woman doing mild exercise had a total metabolism made up of several categories. Let's now change her into a heavy exerciser, which will make most of those categories enlarge and will add some new ones.

First, look at her exercise program. She not only goes to aerobic class three hours per week, which averages about 250 calories per day as previously described, she now lifts weights three hours each week and plays hard tennis for three hours on Sun-

The Subcategories Making Up Metabolism

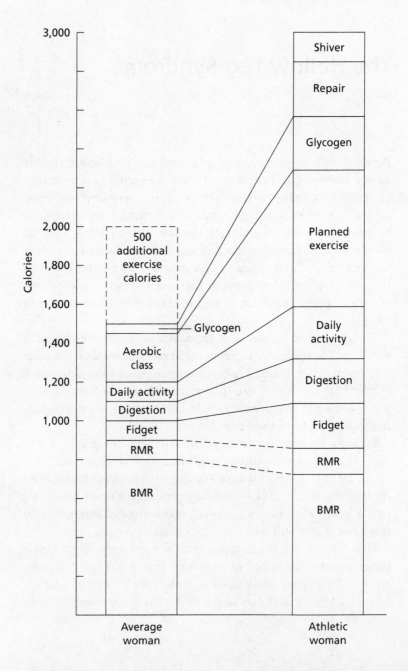

day, burning an additional 500 calories. The numbers are not meant to be exact, but she now burns about three times the number of exercise calories.

Most people, even professionals in the field, would simply add the additional 500 calories to the left side of the graph. They would, as the dotted line shows, expect this woman to now be able to eat 2,000 calories without gaining weight. They're wrong. She can, in fact, probably eat 2,500 calories without gaining weight, and 3,000 is possible. To get a more correct picture of the effects of that extra exercise, look at the bar on the right side of the graph, basically an exploded view of the bar on the left.

> **Fitness buffs have it backward —**
> **exercise *lowers* metabolism.**

Her basal metabolic rate may be higher or lower or may not change at all. It doesn't really matter, because the rise in all other categories is what makes the difference. In my graph I made BMR and RMR a little lower just to illustrate that even a decrease in the resting/basal metabolism in very fit people won't affect their gross need for calories.

Such fit people are always doing something. Even reading a book is interrupted with side trips to check the stove, see who is in the driveway, and other nonessentials that they are not aware of and that our average woman would have avoided. Our average woman may have fidgeted. But our heavy exerciser fidgets a lot.

Heavy exercisers can eat more and therefore digest more. All their calorie-burning digestive processes are geared up, so they can eat even more, significantly increasing their digestion metabolism.

The exercise of daily activities is much greater. These are the people who play Frisbee at the beach while their average friend sits on a blanket. They jump into a volleyball game because it's easy for them. They don't even call it exercise! If asked about yesterday's exercise, they remember only the hour at the health club, forgetting to mention the Frisbee game and three hours of dancing. They not only do more of such activity, they do it more strenuously. In films taken surreptitiously of people playing basketball or soccer or tennis, the fitter ones move more quickly and more often for a given maneuver.

The category of calorie consumption called glycogen is greatly enhanced in heavy exercisers. The dozens of calorie-demanding mechanisms which occur after exercise to get ready for the next exercise are all increased (see "How Dieting Slows You Down," page 68).

And, finally, there are a couple of new categories, repair and shivering, that probably don't occur in the "average" person. Only in hard exercisers do we find the need for actual muscle repair after exercise. And hard exercisers don't bundle up so much when they play in the snow. Instead of putting on extra sweaters and jackets when they get out of the car, they prefer to shiver and spank their hands, warming up the high-calorie way.

In short, even though our new high-exercise woman has added only 500 calories to her planned daily exercise, her metabolism has gone up by 1,000 calories or more.

Adults often feel that they are exercising more and eating less than when they were kids. They may be right about the eating, but are they really exercising more? Perhaps they have more planned exercise, but their unplanned activity has dwindled. They're proud of their thirty-minute jog in the morning, but what are they doing the other twenty-three and a half hours? They blame their weight gain on "getting older," when in fact they just *did* more when they were young. They used to play basketball with the gang, jump on a bike to go to the store, dance all night. Now that they're older they carefully count and record each minute spent exercising. They eat sensible portions of food at well-regulated intervals. They sleep the required eight hours. They do everything "right" — and they gain weight.

The high number of calories that heavy exercisers burn up — their elevated metabolism — is not the result of elevated BMR or RMR, nor does it represent the calories used during their planned exercise. Rather, it is the result of all the other metabolic consequences of heavy exercise.

Don't bug your doctor about your metabolism anymore.

Don't "woe is me, my metabolism is low" anymore.

Don't expect a diet to solve anything.

Don't go to a nutritionist hoping for pills, special diet tricks, or secret formulas to alter your metabolism.

INSTEAD

Look at all the categories that make up metabolism, then think of all the special metabolisms that are inside each category. Which of those hundreds of metabolisms is depressed inside you so that you get fat? You don't know — and no one can tell you. But it doesn't matter now — because you know how to fix them all.

Are You a Mercedes or a Pinto?

Can you remember the old days when even smart people smoked? It was easy to find a cigarette-smoking doctor who would tell you that smoking wasn't all that bad, that the anti-smoking research wasn't conclusive.

Well, if you hate exercise, find a fat doctor. He will probably tell you that exercise isn't what it's cracked up to be, that more research is needed.

Why is it that Doubting Thomases always show up to contest what's obvious, just in time to dampen progress? We all instinctively knew smoking was bad years ago, but the surgeon general wasn't convinced until 1973. The tobacco interests were so powerful that he had to wait for incontrovertible proof before he could state the obvious. In a similar vein, today our government is looking for better ways to spend money on sick people rather than spending money on ways to make people not sick.

The surgeon general could have pulled a fast trick on the pro-smoking people. He could have printed on cigarettes, "There is absolutely no proof that smoking is good for you." Or how about this, "There is absolutely no proof that smoking while pregnant will produce a healthy baby." Print that on cigarette packages and let the tobacco companies try to refute it.

If you are one of those physicians who is still skeptical of the medical benefits of exercise, show us your research.

Can you prove that out-of-shape people live longer or have any medical advantages?

Can you prove that people with thick, unexercised blood are more likely to survive a heart attack?

Can you prove that people with insulin-insensitive muscles are less susceptible to diabetes?

Can you prove that the stress hormones have less damaging effects on out-of-shape people?

Some of us are going to exercise now so that we can have fun when we are eighty. We aren't going to wait for the surgeon general to approve it.

Years ago, when fluoride was shown to prevent tooth decay, change hit the dental profession like an explosion. The use of fluoride in drinking water, toothpaste, and applications by dentists has decreased cavities by 85 percent, one of the miracles of our century. Dentists might well have kept the information to themselves to protect their incomes, but they didn't. As true professionals, they urged a remedy that threatened their own pocketbooks.

Now our physicians are faced with a similar challenge. They, too, have a new miracle pill. My doctor has a sign in his waiting room:

> If exercise could be packaged in a little pill,
> I would give it to every patient.

If everyone became fit, doctors would be looking for patients. There is no question that this "pill" is effective. The question is, will physicians be professional enough to use it?

Let's stop asking foolish questions such as, "Does exercise make people live longer?" That's the stuff of cheap journalism, making headlines that are here today, gone tomorrow. Yes, some research shows that fit people live longer, but other research refutes it. The real question is, "Can I live better?" not "Can I live longer?" Let's not dwell on the few people who live past one hundred. Let's focus on the fat, overweight, out-of-shape people who fill the hospitals.

Let's focus on those average people who, when they were young, felt that nothing was wrong with their bodies, that they were healthy. But their bodies weren't really healthy like an athlete's body. It's a bit like comparing a Ford to a Mercedes. When the Ford is new it may cruise just as well as the Mercedes. Its owner may feel that sharp looks and high performance aren't important. But the Mercedes body has better lungs and a longer-lasting heart behind its higher performance.

It's too bad the health benefits of exercise aren't obvious until we are old. The thin blood produced by exercise moves so easily that even an older, weaker heart can handle it. The extra red blood cells produced by exercise carry so much oxygen that an eighty-year-old can ski at Aspen. When your body has 75,000 miles on it, you're going to wish you had exercised it, as an athlete does, giving it Mercedes qualities.

In the beginning of this book, I told you about my King Muscle pills. It only takes thirty minutes to swallow them, and they'll improve your fitness and health more than any drug ever invented. But I must warn you — beware of the side effects! You'll lose body fat rather quickly. You'll develop an itch to get out and play more often. You'll sleep fewer hours. You'll tend to have memory lapses about minor problems. These pills depress your heart rate and blood pressure. Plus the pills can be expensive; you'll need to budget more for food and new clothes: your appetite will increase while your clothing size shrinks.

I'd like to market these pills, make a fortune, and retire, but the only people who would buy them are the people who have read this book. And if you have read this book, you already have them, don't you?

Index